BabySafe in Seven Steps

BabySafe in Seven Steps

The babyganics® Guide to Smart and Effective Solutions for a Heathly Home

Kevin Schwartz and Keith Garber

The "Founding Fathers" of babyganics®

With Samantha Rose

Ballantine Books Trade Paperbacks
New York

The information and advice presented in this book are not meant to replace or substitute for the advice of your family's physicians and other trained health care professionals. You are advised to consult with health care professionals with regard to all matters pertaining to you and your family's health and well-being.

As of press time, the URLs displayed in this book link or refer to existing websites on the Internet. Neither Random House LLC nor the authors are responsible for, nor should they be deemed to endorse or recommend, any website other than their own, or any content available on the Internet (including without limitation, any website, blog post, information page) that is not created by Random House LLC or the authors, respectively.

A Ballantine Books Trade Paperback Original

Published in the United States by Ballantine Books,
an imprint of Random House,
a division of Random House LLC, New York,
a Penguin Random House Company.

BALLANTINE and the HOUSE colophon are registered
trademarks of Random House, Inc.

LIBRARY OF CONGRESS CATALOGING-IN-PUBLICATION DATA
Schwartz, Kevin.
Babysafe in seven steps: the babyganics guide to smart and effective solutions for a healthy home / Kevin Schwartz, Keith Garber, Samantha Rose.
p. cm
Includes index.
ISBN 978-0-345-54712-5 (paperback)
eBook ISBN 978-0-345-54713-2 (ebook)
1. Child rearing—Safety measures. 2. Home accidents—Prevention.
I. Garber, Keith. II. Title.
RJ61.S393 2014
649'.1—dc23 2014002108

Printed in the United States of America

www.ballantinebooks.com

9 8 7 6 5 4 3 2 1

First Edition

Book design by Diane Hobbing

While we may have outgrown our babyhood, we continue to get nurturing, love, and support so we can thrive . . . and are incredibly lucky to be surrounded by people who do just that. This book is for them.

To our wives, Ali and Nicole, and to our children, Tyler, Ryan, Zachary, Skylar, and Ashton. You keep us inspired, excited, and motivated to dream big.

And of course to our parents, Ellen and Sharon and Seymour, who were the very first to provide us with models of safe, healthy, and happy homes.

Foreword

Every new parent knows the feeling. You come home with your impossibly tiny baby and are overwhelmingly aware of his or her vulnerability. Fortunately, the more we learn about our baby's development, the more empowered we are and knowledgeable about how best to protect them and help them thrive.

Keeping your child healthy actually starts in utero. Your baby is most vulnerable during the first trimester, when all his major organs are developing. This is the time to start thinking about making your home baby-safe. Then once you bring her home, the work continues. Babies' large surface-to-body-mass ratio (i.e. lots of skin on a small body) means they truly are more likely than adults to absorb harmful substances from their indoor and outdoor environments. So all of us, from professionals to parents, have a responsibility to educate ourselves about how to create an ideal baby-safe environment and to apply that education mindfully, consciously, and joyfully!

From the moment you make the life-changing decision to bring a baby into your world (or better yet, from the moment you find out he or she is on the way), it's important to start thinking about how you clean, what you eat, and what kind of air you breathe. As an allergist and pediatrician for the past twenty years, I spend as much time talking to parents about the many ways to keep their babies healthy and safe as I do treating kids once they are sick, and the wisdom and practical advice found in this go-to guide are exactly the kind I want all of the parents of my little patients to have. Kevin and Keith have dedicated their lives to creating personal care and household products that give parents valuable peace of mind. With this book, they take the next natural step, advising parents further about healthy lifestyle choices that will have a positive impact on their babies' lives—every coo, smile, crawl, and step along the way. Here's to a baby- safe world!

Morris Nejat, MD
medical director, New York Allergy and Sinus Centers
assistant clinical professor of Pediatrics, New York University Medical School
instructor in Pediatrics, Columbia University College of Physicians and Surgeons
medical director, babyganics

Contents

Foreword vii

What Is Baby-Safe? xi

Step 1: Mommy Detox 3

Glow Naturally 5

Arooma Therapy 14

A Tall Glass of (Clean) Water 22

A Healthy Plate for Two 29

Decorate with Love 41

Step 2: Crib Improvement 59

Chemical Purge 62

Fighting Grime 72

A Safe Germinator 75

Floors to Adore 80
Scrub-a-Tub-Tub 82
Take a Load Off 85

Step 3: Baby Comforts 91
Fine and Handy 92
Kissy Face 101
Bathtub Basics 111
Hiney Helpers 115

Step 4: Safe Play 129
Warning Labels 130
Babes in (Safe) Toyland 138
First Gear 146
An e-Motional Debate 155

Step 5: Eat Healthy and Happy 163
Learn the Lingo 164
A Clean Plate 176
Family Food Fun 185
Mealtime 194

Step 6: Your Fur Babies Matter, Too 205
Clean and Coiffed 206
A Buggy Situation 213
Playful Tips 218
Low-lying Playmates 220

Step 7: A Baby-Safe World 231
Green Your Outdoor Space 232
Dig In 242
Bug Off Naturally! 245
Fun in the Sun 249
Safety = Freedom! 259

Acknowledgments 265
Index 269
About the Authors 281

What Is Baby-Safe?

You see it every hour, every day. Your baby is constantly exploring her world. (Your world!) Touching, tasting, sensing, and discovering the world is his *full-time job.* This early exploration happens in the bath when her eyes light up as she watches with wonder as bubbles pop and she delights in the power of the splash. It happens when your baby picks up a new "toy"—a rock, a Cheerio, a dog brush!—and he discovers it in his own way by touching and, yes, tasting it.

This seemingly random exploration is not only magical and fun to watch, but it's also incredibly important for your baby's physical, mental, and emotional health (have you noticed how freakin' happy each new discovery makes her?). As parents we all want to encourage this natural curiosity and give our babies the freedom to learn, grow, and thrive. To do this, our babies need a safe environment, right? A "baby-safe" environment. Nothing drastic or confining—we're not talking about building a bubble around your new baby. We know as well as you do that you can't insulate your baby from everything. As a parent, you're naturally protective, but you're also realistic, right? You simply want to create a clean and healthy home where your baby can, well, do what babies do! What we're talking about is creating safety not just for safety's sake but for the sake of your baby's *freedom*—the freedom to satisfy his natural curiosity and happy exploration. The reality is that your baby *will* put his toes in his mouth, lick the table, and go out in the sun. She'll get shampoo in her eyes, probably eat out of the dog bowl (at least once!), and play in the mud. Hey, things happen. *Life happens.* We get it. We're parents, too.

Two dads on a mission

We're Kevin and Keith, the founding fathers of babyganics, and we believe passionately in the freedom of babies to be babies. As dads ourselves, we've had the great fortune of seeing the world through our babies' eyes. They experience it so naturally as a wondrous place, full of excitement and novelty, bursting with new opportunities to grow and learn. This 360-degree view of our babies' world has helped us create products to make your world—inside and out, including everything that touches your baby and that your baby touches—as baby-safe and healthy as possible. That's a parent's most important job, isn't it? That's why we think it's our most important job as well.

If you don't already know about our company, forgive us while we (briefly) describe our products. After all, they're also our babies! babyganics is a full line of natural, nontoxic, and effective household and personal care products for every touchpoint in your baby's life. If you're a mom or dad (or soon to be either one), you're likely to run across our products in your favorite baby retailer, neighborhood grocery, or drugstore. We're in the aisles of household cleaning and skincare, sun protection, laundry, and also in the section of the store you probably find yourself more often than anywhere else—diapers! Our products are designed for babies, but honestly, they're just as much for parents; whether they protect, moisturize, nourish, or clean, their most important ingredient is always peace of mind.

Baby-safe = free + happy!

We created babyganics in 2005 when parents were really beginning to wake up to the fact that many of the household and personal care products they were using could actually be harmful to pregnant moms and their babies. We were both new to the marriage and baby scene ourselves and entering that stage of life when all of our good friends were starting families, too. With all the news and information readily available about chemical pollutants, dangerous contaminants, harmful ingredients, and toxic substances in and around our homes, we wondered, and worried: How many of us were using products that we thought were safe, but were actually putting our little ones in harm's way? We'd wash our dishes and wonder about the soap. We'd get out of the tub and worry about the suds. Our parental instincts kicked in big-time and we took it as our fatherly duty to start reading labels and hunting for products that were both effective and safe for our families. We couldn't find anything out there! And this quickly threw us into panic mode, you know, where you start to think that to be a "good" parent you have to be overprotective, hypervigilant, and maybe even a little—obsessed? Oh yeah, we've been there. We imagined the many ways we could build an isolated and protective bubble around our homes. *Lock the doors and seal the windows! Nothing's getting in that'll harm* my *family!* We let our minds run a little wild until eventually we realized that trying to control the uncontrollable (not to mention the unforeseen future) was kind of pointless. It didn't fit with our lifestyles or personalities. Extremism was a little too—*extreme.* It wasn't the way we wanted to parent. Also, this approach didn't seem to be in the best interest of our babies. What we needed were products and smart solutions that would help us to relax and enjoy this next big step in our lives and that would also allow our babies to just . . . be babies! So we decided to take a balanced approach that was less about fear and extremism and more about creating freedom.

We gathered some of the smartest and most enthusiastic experts we could find: a community of researchers, professors, pediatricians, allergists, and specialists in medicine, science, toxicology, and sustainability and created our own line of baby-safe products that were highly effective, safe, and tested for real-life usage.

This meant that they fit into our (and our babies') normal, not-so-extreme lifestyles. We hoped they would give parents *just like us* the power to easily transition from their current products and habits to ones that were healthier and safer without feeling the need to press the family "uh-oh" panic button. We figured if we wanted natural, common sense, and effective solutions that were also affordable, there must be a lot of other parents out there who wanted them, too. Turns out we were right.

Why this book?

Over the years, many of our loyal customers have asked us: Aside from using babyganics products, what can I do to keep my family healthy, clean, and safe? And our answer is, a lot! And no, it doesn't necessarily involve buying more of our stuff. It starts with arming yourself with relevant, up-to-date, and useful information and making a few small, balanced lifestyle shifts that put the health and safety of your baby front and center, helping to create the nurturing, happy environment we all hope to build. By simply understanding more about the water you drink, the air you breathe, the food you eat, and what's in all those plastic bottles stashed under your sink, you can begin to make smarter choices for your babies that'll give you peace of mind and create the kind of freedom from fear that we all want in our lives. If you change just a few of your regular practices when it comes to sun and skin care, cosmetics, how you play with your kids, furnish your home, and groom your dogs and cats, you'll start to see how it's really pretty easy to create an environment that sets your baby free to develop and explore, live in the real world, and enjoy these important early years!

Follow our seven baby-safe steps and you'll learn how to:

- Evaluate your daily habits and start to make more thoughtful and smarter choices even *before* you bring baby home from the hospital
- Rid your home of toxic cleaners and begin making simple shifts to ensure smarter cleaning
- Protect your baby's skin from dryness, sun, and pesky bugs
- Choose baby gear and toys that are 100 percent fun to play with and also safe
- Ramp up your awareness of healthy foods and get your kids excited about eating "clean"
- Keep your cats and dogs looking, smelling, and feeling good—because what you use on your pets definitely comes into contact with your baby
- Be healthy, happy, and free in the real and wondrous world

Some of these things you may already be doing and if so, good for you! Other ideas might be totally new. Either way, don't worry about what you've done up to now. Throw guilt (and the idea of perfection) out with your baby's bathwater. You've done your very best, and tomorrow is another chance to do it all better. As family guys (wives, pets, and five kids between us!), we really do get how hard it can be for parents to make the daily, balanced choices that go into creating a safe, healthy, and happy environment for their babies. Every day we simply do *our* best at home, and at the office we dedicate our time to helping you do yours. Nothing gets us more excited than sharing information and empowering expectant parents, new moms and dads, and growing families to adopt the products and solutions that will make their lives not only easier but also healthier, happier, more relaxed, and *even safer* than they already are.

We're in this together

No doubt you've already done an amazing amount of thinking, discussing, and planning to help create a happy, safe environment for your baby. And together, we will help you do more. Consider *BabySafe in Seven Steps* your partner in this endeavor, your go-to guide to everything we've taken years to learn. In addition to being dads and business partners, we're also what you might call health and wellness "enthusiasts" (OK, *nuts*), and the kind of guys who like scientific research. Geeky? Yeah, we tend to run in those circles, but what can we say? We're into it. And if we can answer some of your concerns, like, "Is it safe? Will it work?" we're thrilled! We're happy to help you make the best choices at a time when you may be feeling overwhelmed (becoming a parent kinda does that!). Whether you're pregnant, a new mom or dad, or chasing after a toddler, you're probably buying and using a boatload of products to keep your house in order. And with all the scary science out there and vague promises like "green," "organic," "earth-friendly," and "pure" slapped on products at every turn, a trip to the store or a simple purchase online can be a bit crazy-making. What do all those labels mean, anyway? The way we see it, you shouldn't need a degree in toxicology or to spend your precious evenings Googling ingredients to make sense of it all. It's easy to drown in all the information. Sure, you want to know what's out there, but what parent has the extra time and energy for that? This is why we've done the work for you, so you don't have to (and maybe get an extra hour's sleep!)

With the same experts who help us develop our babyganics products, and with the help of other like-minded and informed parents, we've written a book that we hope answers all the questions that keep you up at night and dumbstuck in the household cleaner aisle, and provides you with smart solutions that'll quickly make big-time differences in the lives of those you love most. Will it involve a lot of work on your part? Not really. You've already got your hands full, so we've created a manageable set of steps that you can take at your own pace—but still well before your babies take theirs!

Babies first

Before we try, or suggest *you* try a specific product or practice, we always ask the driving question: Is it baby-safe? Meaning, does it put the health and safety of your baby before *anything else*? You see, there are a lot of companies out there marketing directly to parents like you, calling themselves green, natural, safe for the environment, the planet, and therefore (you would assume) safe for *your baby.* But unless you do the research, you might not know that planet-friendly isn't necessarily people-friendly, let alone baby-friendly. That's right. "Green" and "eco-safe" can sometimes be risky for the most precious thing in your life: your child's ten little fingers and ten little toes.

Before we did our homework, it was hard to believe that a green product could be harmful to babies. But it turns out that a tiny, living, breathing being (that would be your baby) is actually a lot more vulnerable than the planet she sits on. You see, our planet's been around for a lot longer, and is a lot bigger and tougher, than a newborn or toddler. Most parents don't realize that many household and personal care products that are safe for the earth can be toxic to people and especially harmful to pregnant moms and babies.

Consider this in the context of the products you use at home: The "earth-friendly" tub and tile cleaner you use to clean your bathroom may not pose a danger to the environment, typically because once its ingredients have been rinsed down the drain, they begin to break down and are relatively harmless by the time they flow into the ground or water. But when that same natural tub and tile cleaner comes into direct contact with your child's skin or is even merely inhaled by her, it may have a less than *natural* effect. Hydrogen peroxide, for example, is a great natural cleaner, but you can also cook raw meat in it. Not exactly something you'd ever want to use near your baby. Or consider bleach, a tried-and-true favorite of many. A Risk Assessment Report (RAR) by the European Union on bleach (sodium hypochlorite) under Regulation EEC 793/93 concluded that this substance is safe for the environment, but it's also highly corrosive to the skin, lungs, and eyes, and can cause chemical burns and ulcerations. Earth-friendly, maybe—baby-friendly, no way!

Of the chemicals found in the average family's home, more than *one hundred* contain ingredients that don't pose a threat to our planet but when touched, inhaled, or ingested, they have been linked to reproductive and hormone disruption, growth issues, allergies, asthma, and psychological disorders like autism, attention deficit/hyperactivity disorder (ADHD), and obsessive-compulsive disorder (OCD) in children. Can you say—Tox-*ick*? Hey, we're all for a healthy planet, but not at the expense of unhealthy babies—and we don't think you should have to choose.

And you don't. Based on all the research we've done and the information we've gathered from our expert team of doctors, specialists, scientists, professors, and informed parents, each product and practice we introduce to you in the pages ahead seeks to put the health and safety of your baby first—and if a product or practice is safe for your baby, it's family-safe, pet-safe, and most definitely *planet-safe,* which makes our approach a win all around.

BabySafe in Seven Steps

Step 1

Mommy Detox

Ready? Set? Taking the first step toward a baby-safe home starts today! You can start to make significant changes that are healthier for your baby as early as conception by evaluating the products you use on your own body and by becoming even more aware of your personal habits. As soon as our wives, Ali and Nicole, discovered they were pregnant, we both became super focused on everything that could affect our babies at this vulnerable stage of their lives. We understood that the outside world with its contaminants and pollutants was a potential threat to our babies in utero because everything Mom is exposed to, her baby is as well. So we started having conversations with our wives and began to consider what we could each do individually and together as parents to reduce exposure and harm, and keep our growing babies as healthy and safe as possible (like a sort of practice run for our homes once our babies were born!).

What we realized pretty quickly was that if you're a soon-to-be mom or dad who wants to create a healthy, clean, and safe environment for your baby, you're smart to start doing better for *yourself.* That is, learn what's healthy, clean, and safe (and what isn't), and begin to make choices and personal lifestyle shifts that help you improve your own health.

For us, in the months before our babies were born, making shifts toward healthier, cleaner, and safer wasn't such a big deal because naturally we *wanted* to do better for ourselves than ever before. We looked down the road—nine months down the road, to be exact—and we recognized the most significant reason to make healthy change—for our babies. The tiny, precious humans we couldn't wait to welcome into the world! Have you had a of moment of clarity like this, too? We figured as much, so as you get ready and set for the arrival of your little one, we'll share with you what we've learned about

- Glowing naturally
- Breathing a little easier
- Drinking clean and safe water
- Eating happily and healthily
- Decorating with love

Glow Naturally

Pregnancy is the perfect time to evaluate your beauty and skincare routine because the skin is your largest organ. Most of us don't often think about the fact that what goes on our skin has the potential to get *under* our skin and into our bloodstream. In the biz, this is referred to as "topical absorption," and it seriously adds up over time, like sun damage. If we got our blood tested today, we'd each likely discover a bunch of nasty toxins that we absorbed through our skin at some point in our lives. Yeah, it's kinda gross, but the not-so-pretty truth is that we live in a world where most of the products we come into contact with carry some level of toxicity that our bodies absorb little by little over the years. This exposure and accumulation can lead to minor and major health problems for you and, if you're pregnant, for your baby, too. It sounds scary, but by making simple product swaps where you replace even *just a few* of your skincare products with safer alternatives (and there are many out there), you can maintain your existing beauty and skincare routine without the ugly side effects.

Take a minute and think about your favorite cosmetics and skincare products. Have you ever read the ingredient list on the back of all those tubes and bottles? If your answer is "Umm . . . sometimes?" or "I've tried and I don't get what I'm reading," you're not alone. Most of us don't know exactly what we're putting on our skin, and those of us who do read ingredient lists (hey, we already admitted we're science geeks) know that you almost do need a degree in chemistry to understand them. *Almost.* We believe you can make safer choices for you and your baby without a textbook; all you need is some basic knowledge (we'll help you!) about the leading toxic offenders.

Whether you're pregnant or already have children, switching from products that contain any of these chemicals is a smart idea.

Kevin and Keith's
NOT-SO-PRETTY List

PARABENS

Where you'll find them: Personal care products like lotion, shampoo and conditioner, shaving and shower gel, spray tan solution, deodorant, and toothpaste. Parabens are used to preserve a product's shelf life; they slow down the growth of mold in your personal care products and your baby's.

Why they're bad news: Parabens can be absorbed through our skin, scalp, and blood and linger in human fat tissue and breast milk. They've been linked to cancer; they've been found inside breast tumors. There's also strong evidence that parabens are endocrine disrupters—gender-bender chemicals that mess with our hormones. Parabens have been linked to early puberty in girls and reduced testosterone levels in boys.

PHTHALATES

Where you'll find them: Body wash, nail polish, lipstick, fragrances and scented sprays, deodorant, hair gel, hand and body lotions, liquid soap, and shampoo. Phthalates also make plastic toys more flexible and soft (more on this later).

Why they're bad news: Phthalates keep hair spray sticky, mascara from running, nail polish from chipping, and they help fragrances linger longer, but numerous U.S. Environmental Protection Agency studies have documented that exposure to phthalates may threaten our reproductive health. Phthalates are also suspected endocrine disrupters.

SYNTHETIC FRAGRANCES

Where you'll find them: Shampoo, lotion, body wash, bubble bath, body spray, and in baby-care products like diapers and wipes. Basically any personal care, household, or cleaning product that's "scented" contains synthetic fragrance.

Why they're bad news: Many synthetic fragrances and perfumes contain phthalates and other toxic chemicals that can concentrate in human fat tissue and breast milk, and have been linked to hormone disruption, allergic reactions, asthma, migraine headaches, and other respiratory and sinus problems. The ingredients in synthetic fragrance formulas are considered proprietary industry "trade secrets" so the actual ingredients do not have to be disclosed. This is why you often just see the word "fragrance" in the ingredient list.

FORMALDEHYDE

Where you'll find it: Shampoo, deodorant, body wash, nail polish, lipstick, hair coloring, and hair-straightening treatments. Also used in wall-to-wall carpeting, area rugs, and in furniture and building materials made from pressed woods (particle board, chip board, etc.).

Why it's bad news: Especially when inhaled, formaldehyde is a toxic chemical linked to nausea, chronic fatigue, dizziness, ear infections, burning eyes, headaches, joint pain, loss of sleep, and can trigger respiratory irritation and asthma. Oh, and—shocker—it's also been linked to cancer.

HYDROQUINONE

Where you'll find it: Skin lightener, anti-aging products, and hair dye.

Why it's bad news: Hydroquinone heightens skin sensitivity by decreasing the production of melanin pigments in the skin, and simultaneously increasing the skin's exposure to UVA and UVB rays. Hydroquinone may also have carcinogenic effects and has been linked to compromised immunity and reproductive health. It may also cause developmental delays in children who are exposed to it.

PETROCHEMICALS

Where you'll find them: Lotion, foundation, lipstick and lip balm, and in products that list paraffin and mineral oil as an ingredient.

Why they're bad news: Petrochemicals are by-products of petroleum (the stuff used in gasoline)! While petroleum is acknowledged by the U.S. Food and Drug Administration as an approved over-the-counter skincare product, it tends to interfere with the body's own natural moisturizing mechanism. This means products with petrochemicals can easily block pores, irritate the skin, exacerbate acne, and actually lead to dryness and chapping. Ever wonder why some lip balms seem to chap, rather than soothe, your lips?

OK. End of the ugly list.

We're really not trying to freak you out (it's only Step 1!). But if you're feeling a tad overwhelmed, understand that we're simply arming you with a working knowledge of some key ingredients that you'd be smart to avoid, so you can begin to make choices that you can feel really good about.

Q: **Dear Founding Fathers,**

I did it. I read the ingredients on the back of some of my favorite cosmetics and beauty products. Ugh. Nearly everything I've been using since high school is potentially harmful to my baby and me. Problem is, if I throw it all out, I won't have anything left to use. I want to be safe, but honestly, I am not a "bare face" type. Help! I need a makeup plan.

Check These Out!

Beautiful Brands

The easiest way to avoid products with toxic and potentially harmful ingredients is to look for brands and products that are labeled "natural," "nontoxic," and "free" of the ugly stuff. Some brand and product lines we love are:

100% Pure (www.100percentpure.com)
BareEscentuals (www.bareescentuals.com)
Belli (www.belliskincare.com)
Earth Science (earthsciencenaturals.com)
Hourglass (www.hourglasscosmetics.com)
Josie Maran Cosmetics (www.josiemarancosmetics.com)
Juice Beauty (www.juicebeauty.com)
Korres (www.korresusa.com)
Suki Skincare (sukiskincare.com)

A: **Dear Cosmetics Queen,**

It's not necessary to throw everything out! Just consider swapping out a few products that will help you avoid some of the more toxic ingredients, like parabens and phthalates. Our feeling is that if you substitute even somewhere between one and three products with a high toxic profile that you use every day for products that are more natural, healthy, and safe, you're doing better than you were yesterday. (And always better than you did in high school!)

We don't claim to be experts on cosmetics (we rely on a knowledgeable team of dermatologists and our savvy wives to help keep us informed), so our advice for you in this department is pretty simple, and yet effective: Shop for products where the ingredient list is short and in a language that's made to be understood. Look for product labels with words like aloe instead of monoethanolamine. That said, as guys who spend all day developing formulas that are as healthy and safe for babies as possible, we can tell you it's very unlikely you will find a line of cosmetic products where the ingredient mix doesn't contain *some amount* of chemicals. And that's okay. You should know that some chemicals actually do good. That's right, not all chemicals are bad news. Take preservatives, for example, used in many skincare products to keep uninvited organisms away—we're talking about microscopic bugs that grow in your product the longer it sits on the shelf. We think that bugs in your and your baby's lotion are kinda gross (wouldn't you agree?), so some amount of preservatives in skincare products are a good idea and we use them in our babyganics products in levels that are perfectly safe to apply topically. As product designers, we consult with leading toxicologists all the time and we've yet to meet one who believes in an all-out ban of chemicals in skincare products. That's extreme, and we're advocates of a balanced approach. Shop around. See what's out there and ask yourself, "What products are available that will allow me to make a safer choice?"

In addition to switching to skincare products that are more natural, healthier, and safer than what you may have been using up until now, consider our smart solutions for hair and nail care.

SMART SOLUTIONS:
Skin, Hair, and Nails

- Choose mineral-based. Switch to makeup lines primarily derived from naturally occurring minerals like mica, tourmaline, and iron oxides. The real benefit of mineral makeup comes from the fact that many leading brands have a long list of ingredients left *out* of their products, including parabens, mineral oil (very different from mineral-based), chemical dyes, and synthetic fragrance.

- Choose water-based. Switch to skincare products like lotions and creams that are primarily water-based rather than based on mineral oil or petroleum.
- Choose plant-based. Switch to skincare products like lip balms and lotions made primarily with plant-based ingredients like shea butter, aloe, or olive, avocado, and argan oils.
- Don't rely on the "organic" label. Just because it's labeled that way doesn't mean all the ingredients are organic, nor is there an agreed-upon definition from the cosmetics industry as to what organic is. The label can be misleading, so carefully read through the ingredient list *even if* something is certified as organic by the U.S. Department of Agriculture (USDA). Also know that just because something is labeled organic doesn't necessarily make it the most effective or safe. In some cases, organic ingredients can be toxic or allergenic to pregnant women.
- Drop the scents. Synthetic fragrances and perfumes can contain phthalates and other toxic chemicals that can concentrate in human fat tissue and breast milk. Look for products that are labeled "fragrance-free," "phthalate-free," or "unscented."
- Clean your brushes. According to our wives, cleaning makeup brushes tends to be something most women overlook, yet it is one of the most important things you can do! Makeup brushes can be a breeding ground

for bacteria. Regular cleaning with a natural soap and water is an effective and easy way to remove old makeup, oil, dirt, and gunk.

- Go polish-less. Many brands contains formaldehyde, phthalates, and other toxic solvents that can cause nose, throat, and eye irritation (and in high doses damage reproductive health), so either take a nine-month break from your mani/pedi routine or purchase and bring your own "nontoxic" polish to a salon with good air circulation.
- Skip the color. Most doctors recommend either switching to plant- and mineral-based product lines or skipping hair color entirely while you're pregnant. Many hair dyes contain lead acetate (linked to birth defects) and coal tar (linked to cancer), which can pass through your scalp and on to your baby. But since the research is inconclusive, we'll just say that the less you dye your hair, the less you and your baby are exposed.
- Take an honest look in the mirror. Ask yourself, "Do I really need it?" If the cosmetic or skincare product in question is one you're willing to part with (at least until you stop breast-feeding), then we suggest taking a better-safe-than-sorry approach and putting it back on the shelf.

According to Kevin . . .

When my wife, Ali, was pregnant, she didn't want to give up her makeup routine (not that she needs it, if you ask me). But a little makeup makes her feel good—more beautiful in her own skin—so she found suggestions online to help create a new healthier and safer beauty routine, like using organic coconut oil as a body moisturizer and olive oil as a conditioning hair treatment. She became like the MacGyver of better, safer beauty alternatives. I came home one day to find Ali and a group of other mommies-to-be in our front room, soaking their hands in organic milk and applying phthalate-free polish. Women after my own heart!

Arooma Therapy

The importance of breathing fresh, clean air during pregnancy seems obvious, but guess what? Most of us spend our time indoors with the windows sealed shut, recirculating the same old stale, and sometimes toxic, air. Believe it or not, the average American spends approximately 90 percent of their time indoors, and while most people are aware that outdoor air pollution can damage their health, many don't realize that indoor air pollutants can damage it more! According to the EPA, indoor air pollution has been ranked among the top five environmental risks to public health. Here's why: The air in our homes is often a concentrated mix of airborne particles and dust that, depending on factors like chemicals in your cleaning supplies, pollutants in the paint on your walls, synthetic carpeting, and VOC off-gassing (we'll discuss VOCs in detail later), is potentially harmful. Did you know the indoor air you and your baby breathe may be two to five times—and occasionally more than one hundred times—more polluted than anything you'll inhale outside? Whether you live in the High Sierras or Soho, the air outside is generally safer than what's in your home. Most new, updated, and renovated living spaces have been designed to be energy efficient—that is, well sealed—which saves money on our monthly gas and electric bills, but the downside is that when indoor air has nowhere to go, our air quality suffers.

So what does this have to do with babies? Well, in proportion to their weight, babies breathe twice as much air and at a much faster rate than adults. They also breathe through their mouth more, which means they take in more unfiltered toxins and pollutants than we do, and their little bodies aren't able to metabolize and detoxify as quickly and easily as our grown-up bodies. Asthma, an inflammation of the airways that results in less airflow to the lungs, affects up to 7 million children. Bottom line: Your baby needs fresh, clean air, and lots of it, as he crawls and eventually toddles with all his boundless curiosity and energy.

Exhale. Whew. It's going to be OK.

Exposure to a little stale air will not permanently damage you or your baby. Plus, there are a handful of simple solutions that'll make a big impact so everyone can breathe a little easier.

Air it out!

Especially in the early months of your baby's life, we recommend opening your windows for just a few minutes each and every day to flush out the air that's collected inside your home. While we agree that it's better to "air out" when it's nice outside, even when it's chilly or hot we suggest opening your windows and doors to let air pollutants out and invite the clean stuff in. This is one of the simplest and smartest ways to ensure clean and healthy air is getting into your lungs and your baby's lungs.

In most cities, smog and air pollution is typically highest from midafternoon to early evening, generally between 3:00 P.M. and 6:00 P.M. when temps are at their hottest, so if you happen to live next to a congested highway or near a business or facility that pollutes the air, consider waiting until the evening, when the outside air is at its cleanest, to open your windows and doors. For pregnant women especially, we suggest flushing the air out of your bedroom as often as possible and cracking your windows overnight so that the air you breathe while you sleep is clean and fresh.

According to Keith . . .

One night a few years ago my wife, Nicole, and I woke up to what sounded like a seal barking in the other room. It turned out to be our then-seven-month-old Skylar coughing with the croup. We called our pediatrician expecting she'd call in a late-night prescription to the pharmacy, but instead she prescribed such a simple remedy we were skeptical: take Skylar out into the fresh air for a few minutes even though it was 30° F! Nicole and I looked at each other. *Really?* But Sky was so miserable we decided to give it a try. Almost instantly she could breathe more easily. No more coughing. It turned out that a healthy dose of fresh air helped open up her swollen airways. We took her back inside and easily put her down for the night. It's in moments like these that you recognize just how vulnerable your kids are and how simple, common-sense remedies can make a big difference.

Since you can't move the family out and camp on the lawn (at least not every night!), you might want to consider the following smart solutions for maintaining fresh and safe indoor air on a regular basis.

SMART SOLUTIONS:
Freshen Up

- Crack your windows for a few minutes each day to flush out the air that's collected inside your home.
- Check your vents. Periodically check that your clothes dryer, gas stove, heaters, and fireplaces are ventilated correctly. Not sure what "correctly" means? Check out YouTube for helpful how-to videos.
- Get your ducts in a row. Once a year, clean your air ducts and furnace filters, which collect dust and mold.
- Install carbon monoxide (CO) detectors outside bedrooms if you use gas or oil heat or have an attached garage, and check the batteries twice a year.
- Maintain your heating and air-conditioning units yearly. What most people don't know is that the majority of home heaters and air conditioners or cooling systems do not bring fresh air into the house; they

simply *recirculate your indoor air*, so changing out your air filters is key to maintaining high-quality indoor air. This is often a free service so take advantage of it.

- Install working smoke detectors throughout the house and test them monthly.
- Consider installing ceiling fans to maximize ventilation and airflow throughout your home.
- Test for radon. This is an odorless, tasteless *radioactive* gas that is one of the leading causes of lung cancer deaths each year. Radon comes from the natural decay of uranium that is found in nearly all soils. It can travel into your home through cracks or holes in the foundation, where it can build up over time.
- Decorate your living space with plants. Plants absorb toxic, stale air and produce healthy, pollutant-free air. Placing plants around your home is not only affordable; it's also the most natural and efficient way to breathe more safely and easily.

Minimize the stink

High-quality, clean air in your home has another added benefit: It smells better! (Not that we're suggesting your home stinks.) Make a regular practice of cleaning your ducts, vents, changing your heating and AC filters, and cracking your windows from time to time, and, like magic, odors will be reduced!

Q: **Dear Founding Fathers,**

What's the deal with scented candles and air fresheners? I've always used a plug-in that smells like white linen. I've loved this scent for as long as I can remember, but soon after I became pregnant, I couldn't stand the smell. It was the weirdest thing, but it really did start to make me feel nauseous, and eventually I pulled them all out and threw them away. If the smell is making *me* feel sick, could the scent be affecting my baby?

A: **Dear Fed Up with Fake Fresh,**

You're feeling sick for a very real reason. It's the fake scent! Synthetic scents, fragrances, fresheners, and scented candles are often a complex cocktail of toxic ingredients that may cause migraines, allergic reactions, asthma, and other respiratory and sinus problems. (And remember, fragrance manufacturers don't have to disclose the ingredients in their products, so you'll never really know what's in them.) It's safe to assume that your synthetic white linen plug-in isn't safe for you or your baby, so you have our permission to ditch it. "Fragranced" products are now listed as a common source of indoor air and environmental pollution, and the EPA states that the use of synthetic fragrances should be minimized. Contrary to what we may have been led to believe, fresh does not smell like a fake mix of snowflake and pine, a new car, or a citrus grove. If it smells unnatural, it probably is. Our opinion is that the fragrance industry has done a really good job of teaching us to ignore the quality of fresh air. Think about what fresh air really smells like. Nothing! Ahhhhh.

The most important lesson here is that when it comes to determining the cleanest choices for you and your baby, you can't go wrong when you listen to your body (especially if it feels sick).

Helpful Resource: RIFM and IFRA

The fragrance industry is self-regulated but it has at least two organizations in place with a nose for sniffing out dangerous ingredients in fragrance products. RIFM (The Research Institute for Fragrance Materials) tests, evaluates, and draws conclusions on the potential risks and toxicity of fragrance ingredients from which IFRA (The International Fragrance Association) puts safety standards and guidelines into place. Visit their respective sites at www.rifm.org and www.ifraorg.org for the latest news, research, and findings.

According to Keith . . .

When my wife was pregnant she developed a freakish sense of smell. It literally happened overnight. One morning early on in her pregnancy, Nicole—who never misses her morning cup of dark Italian roast—woke up, got a whiff of the coffee brewing in the kitchen, and groaned from the bedroom, "Ugh, get that out of the house!"

We all know that when women get pregnant their taste buds change, but their sensitivity to smells shoots *off the charts.* We say, follow your nose! Nature has a really good way of telling you what's healthy and safe for your baby and what's not.

According to Kevin . . .

Once I got rid of all fake scents in our house, I became extra sensitive when I ran into them outside my home. Like the day I jumped into a cab at JFK airport and noticed it smelled like a vanilla factory. It was overwhelming. After a few minutes I had a physical reaction to the air freshener and started choking. My nostrils felt like they were on fire! I rolled down both backseat windows and stuck my head out like my Lab likes to do. The cab driver shot me a look in his rearview mirror like I was crazy, but I'm all about pure, unscented fresh air now. Anything else completely turns me off. (I make an exception for the smell of hot dogs in the bleachers!)

As a general rule, we think fragrance-free is the safest way to go. Still, we get that sometimes you may want a little something to freshen up a room. We understand that tiny babies have a way of creating their own special "fragrance." When your adorable baby makes a stink, don't just mask the odor with harsh chemicals and pollutants. Consider spritzing with a natural, neutralizing freshening spray. Look for products with no harsh pollutants, free of parabens, sulfates, and phthalates (try our babyganics Fabric and Nursery Freshening Spray). Or consider burning an all-natural soy, palm, or beeswax candle. We like GoodLight natural candles. These products will naturally minimize smells without harming you or your baby. Another alternative for attacking a deep stink is to open a box of tried-and-true baking soda in key spots throughout your home, like in the fridge and under your sinks. Also, sprinkle it on fabrics, car seats, and strollers (but not when your child's in them!) to neutralize and absorb bad odors. It really works. Some disposable diaper pails even include a baking soda release mechanism. Smart designing! By using these natural alternatives you can breathe more easily knowing that your baby can inhale deeply and freely without harm to her delicate lungs.

A Tall Glass of (Clean) Water

Whether it's water for drinking, mixing with formula, cooking with, or bathing in, clean water is always a central part of your family's health. According to the Agency for Toxic Substances and Disease Registry (ATSDR), children in the first six months of life drink *seven times* as much water per pound of body weight as average adults. (No wonder they go through so many diapers!) The good news is the American water supply is pretty darn clean and a big reason for this is that the EPA and the U.S. Department of Health and Human Services have strict regulations that limit the levels of contaminants like viruses, bacteria, pesticides, and radioactive and chemical by-products in our public water. Most of us can assume that our tap water is safe to drink. Still, as water travels over and through the ground, a number of things can happen.

Not to worry. There are many smart solutions you can adopt to make sure your water is free of harmful contaminants and as clean as possible.

SMART SOLUTIONS:
Clean Water

- Let it flow. Run cold tap water every morning for a minimum of thirty seconds to two minutes to flush out the pipes. This will push out any lead or harmful sediment that's collected there overnight.
- Use cold water. Harmful contaminants are more likely to leach into hot water so use a fresh supply of cold water to drink, prepare food with, and mix formula bottles.
- Keep it clean. Unscrew your faucet aerators (that little nob at the end of the spout) and clean the screens on a regular basis.
- Get schooled. Contact your local water supplier and ask for the Annual Water Quality Report. You can almost always find this report online and often a hard copy will arrive along with your bill. It will tell you exactly where your water's coming from and how it's been treated, along with full disclosure of any radioactive, biological, inorganic, and volatile organic or synthetic organic contaminants it's been tested for, and any amounts that have been found.
- Self-test. If after reviewing your local water quality report you're still not satisfied, test your own water supply. Take a trip to your local home improvement store where you'll probably find several water-testing kits to choose from. Whichever kit you buy, the EPA recommends sending

samples to a certified lab for analysis; a list of labs in your area is available from your state or local drinking water authority.

- Filter. If your water exceeds the federal standard for any harmful contaminant—especially lead—consider investing in a water filtration system. If you can budget for it, we recommend purchasing a home unit that filters for chlorine, lead, bacteria, high levels of fluoride, and other contaminants throughout your entire house. Our opinion is that if you're living in an area where the tap water is at all suspicious, it doesn't make sense to filter only the water at your kitchen sink. Plus, a full home-filtering system requires less maintenance overall than replacing individual filters throughout the house.
- Protect your ground water. If you drink from a well and live close to farmland, an industrial plant, or a gas station, it's a smart idea to have your water tested once a year for bacteria and contaminants.

Q: **Dear Founding Fathers,**

My husband and I have a bet. I say the water that comes out of our fridge is safer to drink than the water coming from our unfiltered tap. It definitely tastes better, so I assume it's also safer. He says it's the same. Who wins?

A: **Dear Fresh from the Fridge,**

You can probably declare yourself the winner of this round. Almost all refrigerators made in the last decade include a water filter, making what's coming out of your fridge dispenser healthier and safer than what's coming from your tap. So now, the only thing to be cautious of is the indicator light. A red light means your filter is spent. Change it! Also, when the flow of water starts to slow down, when it seems like it takes *forever* to fill up a glass, your filter's probably gone bad. Change it! When filters aren't properly maintained, they can not only release contaminants into your water, but they can create and grow their own bacteria. So, since you won the bet, make your husband change the filters!

Kevin and Keith's
NOT-SO-CLEAN List

LEAD

Where you'll find it: Mostly in water, pipes, dust, and paint in pre-1978 homes. Can also be found in PVC plastic, costume jewelry, metal toys, and porcelain. Lead is also frequently found in outdoor soil and at renovation sites.

Why it's bad news: Lead is a well-known toxin and, according to the EPA, it is particularly dangerous to pregnant women and babies. Lead exposure can result in miscarriage or premature birth and can also impact the health of your baby's developing bones. Once outside the womb, babies are at a high exposure rate to lead because they're more apt to touch or put objects that contain lead from dust or soil in their mouths and ingest it. Babies' developing brains and nervous systems are more sensitive to the damaging effects of lead. Learning and hearing problems, lower IQ, slowed growth, and anemia have been linked to lead exposure. In adults, lead can decrease kidney function and increase blood pressure. All in all, lead is bad news.

Beginning in January 2014, changes to the Safe Drinking Water Act will further reduce the maximum allowable lead content in pipes and plumbing fittings and fixtures. For further steps you can take to minimize your exposure, go to http://www2.epa.gov/lead.

Be tap-happy!

Seriously, though, you can relax. As we said earlier, the American water supply is pretty darn clean. A report by Food and Water Watch, a non-profit organization that advocates for policies that will result in access to safe and affordable drinking water, found that well over 90 percent of our tap water is safe on a state and federal level, so chances are very good that the water out of your home tap is perfectly safe for drinking, mixing with formula, cooking with, and bathing in. You probably don't need to change a thing, unless, that is, you've been avoiding the tap and drinking bottled water instead. Yeah. Read on.

Whether it's from Whole Foods or your corner market, bottled water (no matter how expensive or big the brand) does not have to adhere to the same health and safety standards and strict guidelines, nor does it have to be tested as frequently, as your local tap water. The most recent tests by the Natural Resources Defense Council (NRDC), a New York City–based, non-profit, non-partisan international environmental advocacy group, indicate that bottled water isn't any safer than tap water. In fact, as illogical at it sounds, a lot of times it's *less* safe. As the federal bottled water standards are generally pretty weak, sometimes bacteria, excessive fluoride, and—in more than a few cases—arsenic has shown up in our bottled water. So if you've been thinking all along that bottled is better, get tap-happy.

Filtered tap water is not only healthier, but also much cheaper than bottled water. In California, tap water costs around $0.001 per gallon, while bottled water is $0.90 a gallon. We're not mathematicians, but even we can recognize that tap water is significantly less expensive than bottled water! Tap water is also a whole lot less wasteful. Did you know that if you stacked all of the water bottles purchased in New York alone, they would reach the moon? No kidding. As we understand it, U.S. landfills are overflowing with two million tons of trashed water bottles, and these bottles take a long time (like, one thousand years) to biodegrade, and if incinerated they produce toxic fumes. Plus, the amount of fresh water used to produce the bottles far exceeds the actual drinking water inside them. Yep, it's estimated that three liters of water is used to package one liter of bottled water. Gulp. You do the math this time—it's incredibly wasteful. Finally, when you get your recommended six to eight glasses of water a day from a plastic bottle, you significantly increase your chances of ingesting a mouthful of bisphenol A (BPA), a plasticizer that with extended use, repeat washing, and exposure to heat, can leach nasty toxins out of the plastic. Because of this, many of the big chain stores have stopped carrying and selling plastic bottles that contain BPA.

Since then, many of the plastic manufacturers have stopped making bottles with BPA. But it's still out there, so the easiest way to avoid it is to stop drinking from plastic bottles. We recommend using glass, stainless steel, or ceramic bottles whenever possible, or buying reusable plastic products clearly labeled "BPA-free" to fill up with filtered tap water. Lifefactory glass bottles and Bobble products with built-in filters are popular at the babyganics offices.

Kevin and Keith's
BOTTLE BEWARE List

BISPHENOL A (BPA)

Where you'll find it: Plastic water bottles, sippy cups, pacifiers, baby bottles, plastic toys, and register receipts. Also, BPA can be found in the lining of baby-formula containers and canned goods like soup, fruit, tuna, and vegetables. Recycling code 7 may mean the product contains BPA.

Why it's bad news: The National Institutes of Health has expressed concern that exposure to BPA affects brain and neurological development in fetuses, infants, and young children. It's also a suspected endocrine disrupter that may interfere with hormonal development and reproductive growth and it's been linked to breast cancer, prostate cancer, infertility, low birth weight, early puberty, diabetes, and teenage obesity.

A Healthy Plate for Two

If you're pregnant, you're likely drinking more water, not only because you're extra thirsty but also because your doctor probably told you to. You've probably heard, "Drink plenty of water, get lots of sleep, exercise moderately, and eat a diet of lean protein and dairy, fiber, whole grains, and fruit and veggies, and take vitamins and minerals like folic acid and iron. Oh, and cut out the caffeine and alcohol." With five kids between us, our wives have heard the pregnancy spiel many times, with its emphasis on how the health and future of a developing baby is directly impacted by how the mom-to-be treats her body over the next nine months.

Of course, your doctor's right. If you're going to get into habits that are safer for you and your baby, eating clean is one of the smartest and relatively easiest things you can do to make sure you deliver the healthiest baby possible. In the months ahead, your obstetrician will continue to be your best resource when it comes to helping you build a balanced prenatal and postpartum diet that best works for you, your baby, and, hey, even your partner! But based on the research we've done and the personal experiences we've had, we'd like to take a moment now (with a more lengthy discussion in Step 5) to give you a few pointers on how to create a balanced prenatal eating plan that also significantly reduces your exposure to pesticides, bacteria, and other potentially harmful toxins and contaminants in many of the popular foods you buy. We offer these guidelines not so that you feel restricted, but so that, knowing you are safe, you can feel free to eat what you most enjoy!

Detox your produce

We're sure you already know all about the good things that come from packing your prenatal diet with fiber and vitamin-rich fresh fruits and veggies. (Not the least of which is a healthy baby!) But you should know that some produce is actually smarter to eat than others. It's fairly well known that farmers use pesticides and insecticides to protect their crops and increase production. It's true that federal regulations limit the amount of pesticide and insecticide farmers can use on conventionally grown fruits and veggies, and yet the EPA's safety levels aren't always safe. Studies continue to establish the widespread presence of pesticide residue on many of the foods we eat (in government tests analyzed by the EWG, detectable pesticide residues were found on 67 percent of food samples *after* they had been washed or peeled), and at elevated levels that may compromise our health. Pesticides can be toxic to the nervous system, especially for pregnant women, and for babies, whose vulnerable bodies and brains are still developing. Pesticides can affect a baby's birth weight, and compromise a full-term pregnancy.

Still, as far as we're concerned, the benefits of eating fresh produce outweigh the risks. A diet with lots of produce is healthy, obviously, and you can significantly lower your exposure to pesticides and insecticides by avoiding certain fruits and vegetables in favor of safer alternatives. For making the best choices, we turn to the EWG's Shopper's Guide to Pesticides in Produce called the "Dirty Dozen Plus." Based on the organization's most recent research and testing in 2013, the fruits and veggies to avoid, or buy organic, are:

- Apples
- Celery
- Cherry tomatoes
- Cucumbers
- Grapes
- Hot peppers
- Kale and collard greens
- Nectarines (imported)
- Peaches
- Potatoes
- Spinach
- Strawberries
- Summer squash
- Sweet bell peppers

A good rule of thumb is that leafy greens or anything with an edible skin increases your risk of pesticide exposure, and fruits and veggies with a skin you peel off are generally safer. The fruits and veggies lowest in pesticides, what EWG calls the "Clean Fifteen," are:

- Asparagus
- Avocados
- Cabbage
- Cantaloupe

- Corn
- Eggplant
- Grapefruit
- Kiwi
- Mangoes
- Mushrooms
- Onions
- Papayas
- Pineapples
- Sweet peas (frozen)
- Sweet potatoes

So what do you do if, say, you *love* strawberries and buying organic just isn't in your budget? We think you'll like our answer. Eat what you love to eat. Just be smart about it. Lower your exposure as much as possible. If giving up strawberries or reducing your exposure to contaminants by buying organic isn't something you're willing or able to do, then try a few of these smart solutions.

SMART SOLUTIONS:
Reduce Your Exposure to Pesticides

- Buy local produce in season. Be sure to check with your local market or farmer, but generally, local produce is much lower in chemical residue because it isn't traveling far from where it was grown to your kitchen (a fruit grown overseas obviously has a lot farther to travel). Preservatives and chemicals used to stall the ripening process are not necessary, so local produce is typically safer to eat.
- Wash all produce. Lightly scrub with cold water before eating.
- Thoroughly peel fruits and veggies. While this removes much of their natural fiber, it works wonders at removing icky residue.
- Remove the outer leaves. On leafy vegetables like lettuce, kale, and cabbage, remove the outermost leaves where pesticides or residue is more likely to have settled.
- Grow your own. Plant your own organic garden free of pesticides.

Selecting the safest from the sea

You probably don't need us to tell you that fish is good for you. It's just something we should all eat regularly, and it's an especially good choice if you're pregnant—

if you're smart about it. Upside: Fish is low in fat, vitamin rich, and packed with protein and omega-3 fatty acids that help with heart health and the development of your baby's brain. Downside: Eating seafood increases your exposure to methylmercury, which is absorbed by fish as they swim and feed in exposed and polluted rivers, lakes, and oceans. Mercury has been linked to miscarriage and preterm birth, and babies who were exposed in the womb may suffer physical and developmental delays with language and attention, and experience memory problems. So, what do you do—avoid seafood altogether? Not necessarily. The same rule applies to seafood as to produce—minimize your risk.

Learn which fish are safest to eat. While nearly all fish contain some traces of methylmercury, the FDA, EPA, and the Environmental Defense Fund, which promotes sustainable and healthy oceans, recommend choosing fish with the lowest levels of mercury and limiting your consumption to about twelve ounces a week, or two servings. (Eat six ounces or less a week of white albacore tuna and local fish, especially if you are unsure of local water contamination.) When you limit your consumption in this way, you can feel healthy and safe eating these swimmers:

- Arctic char (farmed)
- Butterfish
- Calamari
- Catfish (U.S.)
- Clams (farmed)
- Cod (Pacific)

- Crab (Dungeness)
- Crawfish (U.S.)
- Haddock
- Halibut (Pacific)
- Oysters (farmed)
- Pollack (wild)
- Salmon (wild)
- Sardines (U.S.)
- Scallops (farmed)
- Shrimp (U.S.)
- Tilapia (U.S.)
- Trout (farmed)
- Tuna (canned light)
- Whitefish

As you can see, you have a lot to choose from, but be aware that the FDA is pretty firm about sticking to the "safe" list. While there's a little more wiggle room with produce, when it comes to fish, the FDA recommends that pregnant women, nursing mothers, and children absolutely avoid:

- King mackerel
- Shark
- Swordfish
- Tilefish

The reason bigger fish should be cut out of your diet is because since they have lived longer, they had more time to ingest mercury, and since they feed on fish that feed on fish that have likely also ingested mercury, they have accumulated the contaminant in their bodies. According to the FDA, these fish pose the greatest risk for mercury exposure and should be totally avoided.

According to Keith . . .

Nicole had a horrible second pregnancy: months of morning sickness that lasted all day long. She lived on pretzels, saltines, and animal crackers. She was hardly eating and we were both kind of worried about her nutrition. One day I was at my son's basketball practice when I got a call from Nicole—she was craving tuna salad on a bagel. Even though I was psyched she was hungry, I wasn't really psyched about her craving. Without thinking, I blurted out, "Honey, you know tuna has a lot of mercury." I can't print what she said, but let's just say I'm lucky we're still married. I left my son at practice and drove like a maniac to the nearest bagel shop. So yeah, the lesson here is it's about balance. Nicole's body was telling her (uh, and me) that she needed the protein and maybe the omega-3s. One tuna sandwich wasn't going to hurt, and it was going to make her very *very* happy.

Kevin and Keith's
BAD THINGS IN GOOD FOOD List

PESTICIDES

Where you'll find them: Pesticide residue can attach itself to conventionally grown fruits and veggies. Exposure can also occur through water, soil, indoor, and outdoor air.

Why they're bad news: In children, pesticide exposure has been linked to a variety of health problems, including cancer, endocrine disruption, as well as nausea, muscle weakness, and skin, eye, and lung irritation. Some studies indicate that children who are exposed are at greater risk for neurological problems and delayed brain development.

METHYLMERCURY

Where you'll find it: Mercury occurs naturally in the environment, but when it accumulates in streams, rivers, and oceans, it's turned into methylmercury, which fish absorb and ingest as they swim and feed. Methylmercury builds up in the body over time.

Why it's bad news: A neurotoxin that crosses the blood-brain barrier, it's believed to be harmful to the growing brains of fetuses and young children, leading to language, attention, and memory problems.

POLYCHLORINATED BIPHENYLS (PCBs)

Where you'll find them: PCBs are an industrial waste product that collects in the skin and fatty tissue of fish, especially farmed salmon.

Why they're bad news: PCBs can cross the placenta and contaminate breast milk. They're linked to breast cancer, cognitive loss, endocrine disruption, and behavioral and developmental problems in children.

Pass on the deli tray

It's a pity but true: a lot of soft cheeses, lunch meats, and things like pâté and sashimi from the market or gourmet deli are not an ideal choice for you and your growing baby. Here's why: A bacterium called listeria monocytogenes thrives in cold temperatures and when you eat foods contaminated with it, it can lead to listeriosis, a rare but serious disease that can infect the placenta and amniotic fluid and can cause miscarriage, stillbirth, and premature birth, or infection in your newborn. We know it sounds super scary, but it can be easily avoided.

SMART SOLUTIONS:

Bac(teria) Off!

- Avoid unpasteurized milk. This includes cow and goat. Also skip unpasteurized cheese, specifically soft cheeses like Brie and Camembert and Mexican cheeses like queso blanco. Choose instead pasteurized cheese like ricotta and cream cheese and hard cheeses like Parmesan and cheddar. Cultured dairy products like yogurt are typically safe, but if you're in doubt, read the label first to make sure they're made with pasteurized milk.
- Stay away from cold cuts, refrigerated pâtés, and refrigerated smoked or pickled fish unless they're cooked until steaming hot. Avoid prepared salads, especially those containing eggs, chicken, or seafood.
- Skip raw foods like eggs and sushi.
- Cook meat, poultry, and fish till done! Most meat should be cooked to a temperature of 160° F. If you don't have a food thermometer to test the internal temperature of meat, cook it until it's no longer pink in the middle and resist sneaking a sample before it's done.
- Heat up those leftovers. Because listeria contamination can also occur after food has been cooked and the bacteria can survive and grow in the fridge, heat all previously cooked leftovers to 165° F or until they're steaming hot.
- Avoid contaminating food. Keep uncooked meat, poultry, or seafood

separate from clean produce and from cooked food. This means separate plates and cutting boards.

- A clean kitchen is a safe kitchen. Wash counters, cutting boards, dishes, utensils, sponges, and your hands with hot soapy water after you've touched potentially contaminated food and before you handle clean food.

Helpful Resource:
Can I Eat It?
What's safe to eat during pregnancy? Parenting.com's pregnancy diet and nutrition app is a great resource for moms-to-be on what's safe and healthy to eat during pregnancy, and includes insights into fish and dairy products, produce, beverages, "superfoods," and more. Download the app at the iPhone App Store.

According to Kevin . . .

For my wife, Ali, going mostly organic and reducing how much seafood she ate while she was pregnant and breastfeeding wasn't really a big deal. She switched to foods that were healthier and safer when she could and avoided the rest. One night when we were out to dinner I decided to put in my two cents. I suggested she might also want to pass on her beloved cheese plate. I don't remember her exact words, but it was probably along the lines of Nicole's reaction to Keith's suggestion that she skip the tuna. Let's just say she had her cheese.

Both Keith and I discovered the hard way how our wives became pretty exhausted (nine months is a long time) feeling like they had to be hypervigilant and super-careful every time they ate a meal, and face judgment if they didn't automatically pass on their favorite foods. If you're feeling this way, too, try looking at it this way—the whole point of eating healthier and adopting safer solutions is to feel freer to enjoy your pregnancy, not to feel more constricted!

Decorate with Love

OK, enough about the kitchen. Let's head into the nursery. Here's your excuse for not having set yours up yet: You were just waiting for some guidelines. We're here to help!

Oh, yeah, we've been there. We get that decorating the baby's nursery can be exciting and fun but also (OMG!) overwhelming and never ending. For us, scoping out all the baby gear on the market was like learning a new language. Between the WubbaNub, the Woombie, and the Boppy pillow, there is so much stuff and "friendly advice" out there it's easy to become convinced that *you gotta have it all*! We say focus on the basics. Decorate simply and purchase only what you need (trust us, you can count on grandparents and childless aunts and uncles to go nuts with the rest). By taking a minimalist approach, you'll stay sane, but also you'll be limiting your baby's exposure to potential irritants found in many baby products and nursery furnishings. Did you know the average American nursery contains hundreds of chemicals that threaten your baby's air quality? Don't gasp. We'll help you bring that number *way* down.

Start with the walls

Check This Out!
Non-VOC Paints
There are many no to low-VOC interior paints available made from natural raw ingredients, such as plant oils and resins, milk casein, and natural latex, offering you baby-safer alternatives to many of the traditional toxic offenders. Here's a sampling of some we like and recommend:

- **Green Planet Paints (www.greenplanetpaints.com)**
- **Benjamin Moore Pristine Eco Spec Paint (http://www.benjaminmoore.com)**
- **Anna Sova wall paint (www.annasova.com)**
- **Yolo Colorhouse (http://www.yolocolorhouse.com)**
- **Lullaby Paints (http://lullabypaints.com/)**
- **Harmony Interior Acrylic Latex (http://www.sherwin-williams.com)**

Look at the nursery walls as a blank canvas. (And maybe one that your baby eventually will want to lick?) If you want to brighten or freshen up your baby's space with a coat of fresh paint, OK—go for it. Just be sure to use a water-based paint with low or no volatile organic compounds (VOCs), which you can easily find at your nearest hardware store in all kinds of textures and colors.

Using low- or no-VOC paint is the safest approach. A fresh coat of paint that contains smelly, synthetic VOC fumes can cause respiratory, allergic, and immune complications in utero, in infants, and in children. These fumes can also cause nasal congestion, eye irritation, headache, and nausea in adults, particularly pregnant women. So buy a low- or no-VOC paint and primer and hand the brush over to someone who's not pregnant, as it's really best that pregnant women aren't exposed to paint fumes, period. Send the painters into the nursery two to three months before your due date (which will give the room ample time to off-gas VOCs), make sure the room is well ventilated during the painting process, and once the job is done, close the door and stay out of there for at least a week.

The other thing to think about when it comes to the nursery walls is lead exposure. We talked about the health hazards of lead when we discussed the importance of clean water, and we mention it again here because back in the day (pre-1978) many homes were painted with lead-based paint. If you live in one of these older homes, chances are pretty good that there's some amount of lead in your walls. And do you really want to spend your time pulling your baby's exploring hands away from the walls? Hold on, no need to move out! It's also very likely that over the years, the same walls have been covered up by lead-free paint, wallpaper, or both, creating a protective sealant. Still, relying on layers of paint to protect you is not a real plan. Paint deteriorates, peels, gets dinged, scraped, and chipped, and if any repairs or renovations have been done to your home where walls, windows, or door frames have been sanded or torn down—forget about it. If any lead has been buried, it will now be released as contaminated dust into the air you're breathing.

If you own a home built before 1978 we recommend that you test for lead. You can pick up an inexpensive lead-testing kit at your nearest home improvement store. If you find lead, bring in a certified lead-removal specialist to take care of it. (Don't try to do it yourself!) If you're a renter, it's your landlord's responsibility to provide you with any known information concerning lead-based paint in your building, along with an EPA-approved pamphlet on identifying and controlling lead-based paint. Learn more about your rights at www.epa.gov.

Oh yeah. Floors too.

Walls, check. On to the place where your baby plays, crawls, licks, eats, and rolls around. The floors! VOC gasses can be emitted from carpet also, so if you're thinking of covering your baby's nursery floor with cushy carpeting to protect his or her soft head . . . um, think twice. Wall-to-wall carpet feels good to crawl around on, but most new, synthetic carpets are treated with chemicals in the fibers, dyes, adhesive, and backing material that give off nasty fumes that your babies can easily inhale (remember, they breathe twice as much air as we do). Chemicals from carpeting can cause headaches, dizziness, nausea, and fatigue and interfere with fetal and child development. Also, carpeting traps allergy-producing dust, pet dander, bacteria, mildew, and mold. Gunk like this just loves to collect deep in your carpets, and if that's not enough to turn you off to carpeting, when it comes time to clean, most carpet cleaners contain harsh chemicals that only add to the air-quality problem! Not to worry. As always, there are smarter solutions.

SMART SOLUTIONS:

More on Floors

- Replace old wall-to-wall carpeting with nontoxic materials like hardwood, bamboo, cork, or natural linoleum.
- Throw down a rug. If you want to add a layer of cushioning and a splash

of color to hardwood floors or cover existing carpeting, throw down an easily washable, natural-fiber area rug and underlay. Look for rugs made from natural cotton, sea grass, mountain grass, bamboo, wool, jute, cactus, nettle, and hemp. For the nursery, we also like many of the woodgrain foam play mats. They're cushy and fun.

- Be safe and smart about your cleaning. Rather than kicking up dust, dander and debris with a dry broom or by shaking and beating rugs, try damp mopping with a regular sponge, cloth, or a string mop and a baby-safe, plant-based cleaner.

Q: **Dear Founding Fathers,**

We live in a rental unit with wall-to-wall carpeting. I'd love to pull up the carpeting for the safety of my baby, as you suggest, but don't think our landlord will go for it. What's my backup plan?

A: **Dear Carpet Captive,**

OK, so you can't pull up the rug. Your best backup plan is to just keep the carpeting you have clean and safe. Unless your landlord just put down carpeting, the potential for harmful VOC gases is minimal. Any toxic chemicals that were originally in the carpet are long gone, so just concentrate on keeping your carpeting clean. Vacuum regularly, invest in a high-efficiency particulate air (HEPA) filter (most new vacuums come with one), and remember to clean the filter. Also, open those nursery windows once a day to maintain high air quality.

Natural Zs

You might be sleep deprived for the next few months (uh, years?) but your baby will spend half his or her time—about ten to fourteen hours a day—sleeping. So it's important for you to think about how to make this time safe and healthy, too. While you'll spend a bit more money, we recommend investing in a crib or bassinet mattress made of unbleached, untreated natural fibers and materials such as organic cotton, natural latex, wool, soy, or coconut palm. These materials are a healthier alternative to conventional mattresses that are often chemically treated with things like polyurethane foams and toxic fire retardants.

Kevin and Keith's RESTLESS SLEEP List

VOLATILE ORGANIC COMPOUNDS (VOCs)

Where you'll find them: Volatile organic compounds (VOCs) release as gases and are carried through the air into our noses and lungs. Concentrations of VOCs are consistently higher indoors (up to ten times more!) than outdoors. VOCs are emitted from paints and lacquers, paint strippers, carpeting, rug and oven cleaners, pressed wood and other building materials, and office equipment such as copiers and printers, correction fluids, carbonless copy paper, and glues and adhesives.

Why they're bad news: VOCs are easily inhaled and can cause eye irritation and nasal congestion, headaches, nausea, and vomiting. They are also possibly carcinogenic.

POLYURETHANE

Where you'll find it: The predominant foam filling inside conventional baby mattresses and mattress pads.

Why it's bad news: Polyurethane foam can emit toxic chemicals, including formaldehyde and PBDEs, that, according to the EPA, can cause breathing problems, coughing, asthma, headaches, fatigue, and nausea, as well as skin irritation and allergic reactions. Infants and children exposed to polyurethane may develop reproductive problems, learning difficulties, and memory loss.

POLYBROMINATED DIPHEYNL ETHERS (PBDEs)

Where you'll find them: PBDEs are flame-retardant chemicals (they stop the spread of fire) that can be found in many foam products like carpet pads, crib mattresses, mattress pads, changing-table pads, nursing pillows, car seats, and children's pajamas.

Why they're bad news: When PBDEs break down into airborne dust that's either ingested from hand to mouth contact or inhaled, it can lead to an array of health problems, including reproductive issues like undescended testicles, hormone and thyroid disruption, and delayed puberty. PBDEs have also been linked to cancer. PBDEs build up in our bodies over time and have been detected in breast milk. Studies show that exposure in the womb is associated with low birth weight and neurological impairment, such as learning disabilities and lower IQs. The good news—foam items containing PBDEs were withdrawn from the U.S. market in 2005.

If an organic mattress isn't in your budget (did we mention generous grandparents?), consider buying an organic mattress pad or an organic mattress cover. This may be a more affordable option for you, and a tightly woven organic mattress pad works well as a barrier between the mattress and your baby, trapping any toxic "off-gassing" dust that may be released from the mattress as it breaks down over time. A pad or cover can also help limit exposure to any contaminants in the mattress that could irritate your baby's skin. Another affordable option is a mattress pad made of nontoxic, food-grade polyethylene plastic, which also works as a sealant, reducing exposure to mattress fumes.

Whatever you decide to do, we strongly suggest that any mattress, pad, or fitted mattress pad cover you bring into the nursery be waterproof. (We love organic wool for this reason. It works and it's natural.) Sleeping babies might look angelic, but you'll quickly find that they are great multitaskers, able to drool, spit up, and pee while fast asleep. A waterproof cover protects the mattress from getting wet and becoming a home for bacteria.

Finally, when it comes to sheets, if you've already gone ahead and spent the money on an organic mattress, pad, or fitted cover, you might as well go all the way and put a set or two of natural fiber, unbleached, and untreated sheets into your checkout cart. As far as we're concerned, it doesn't make a whole lot of sense to cover your baby-safe mattress with sheets treated with the very same toxic chemicals and repellents that you've taken steps to avoid. Would you agree? We kinda thought you would, so in addition to switching out your baby's sheets, consider the following smart solutions to ensure an even better night's sleep.

SMART SOLUTIONS:
Safe Sleeping

- Wash all new bedding and sheets in hot water and dry them on hot before using. This helps to remove chemical and manufacturing residue.
- Air new mattresses, pads, and covers outdoors or in a ventilated garage for a few days before putting your baby to sleep on it. When the "new smell" is gone, you'll know it's safe to bring inside.
- Make it a good fit. Your baby's mattress should be the same size as the crib so there are no gaps to trap little arms or legs. If you can fit more than two fingers between the mattress and the side of the crib, it's not snug enough. Rest assured, most baby mattresses are designed to fit a standard baby crib.
- Go bump-less. According to new guidelines released by the American Academy of Pediatrics (AAP), bumper pads should no longer be used in

cribs. Bumpers carry a potential risk of suffocation, strangulation, or entrapment because infants lack the motor skills or strength to turn their heads should they roll into something that obstructs their breathing.

- Let your guard down. Drop-side cribs are now out, too. They also carry a risk of accidental suffocation and strangulation.
- Stay firm. The only thing that should be in the baby's crib is your baby, a mattress, and a sheet. All those fluffy receiving blankets, hand-stitched pillows, and stuffed "loveys" you were given as shower gifts should stay out of the crib . . . for now. Swaddling and sleep sacks are safe (and cozy) alternatives to loose blankets.
- Look for merchandise certified by the Juvenile Products Manufacturers Association. The JPMA seal will assure you that the product conforms to all standard safety, performance, and functionality requirements.
- Refer to the U.S. Consumer Product Safety Commission's Crib Information Center for the most up-to-date regulations and recalls.
- Always, Go Back to Sleep. Always put your baby on her back to sleep to reduce the risk of sudden infant death syndrome (SIDS).

Build a better table

Walls and floors—check! Crib mattress and sheets—double check! Your nursery is almost ready (even if you're not!). Sure, you can decorate *more,* but if you want to keep it simple, stick to the basics and focus on creating a healthy and safe environment that reduces the risk of exposure to toxic chemicals and contaminants.

Now, the changing table. We recommend a sturdy one with a two-inch guardrail around all four sides and a safety strap.

According to Kevin . . .

When we first started using the changing table with Tyler we just couldn't figure out what the strap on the side was all about. It seemed like an overprotective little seat belt. Maybe some babies are wild, but Tyler was pretty chill. But when he got to be about six months old, we got it. This kid was a thrasher! Without that strap he would have wriggled right out of our hands and dropped straight to the floor. The people who build these things are way ahead of new parents. So buckle your baby down. They get new ideas quickly!

In addition to the necessary safety belt, consider what your changing table is made of. Much of the reasonably priced, build-your-own furniture is made from pressed wood, plywood, and particleboard, which usually contain glues and lacquers with formaldehyde—yeah, that nasty chemical and suspected carcinogen we talked about earlier. A lot of furniture manufacturers and retailers like IKEA have made big strides in lowering the formaldehyde emission levels in their wood products.

Still, if you're unsure about the assembly-required crib or changing table that's in forty-five pieces on your living room floor, take matters into your own hands: Once the piece is put together, seal the exposed ends (the scratchy, rough edges that look like unfinished wood) with a nontoxic sealant and move it outdoors to ventilate for a few days. This will really reduce your exposure to unhealthy fumes. Of course, you can always buy natural unfinished wood and finish it yourself with a water-based sealant and stain (but with a baby on the way, who has time for that?).

Finally, when choosing a changing-table pad, think about how the foam pads are often filled with the same polyurethane foam as a lot of conventionally manufactured crib mattresses. So again, if you can budget for one, we recommend investing in a changing pad filled with natural materials, like organic cotton. If that's not an investment you're able to make, let the pad sit outside for several days before bringing it in and consider covering it with a changing-table cover that's made of nontoxic, food-grade polyethylene plastic.

Helpful Resource: Greenguard Environmental Institute

Check out the Greenguard Certification Program. It helps buyers identify products and materials that have low chemical emissions, improving the quality of the air in which the products are used.

Almost done. There's just one more thing to think about—for now—and that's windows. The most important thing to remember when it comes to window safety is keeping those hanging window cords away from your baby's fingers. His curious hands will want to grab, pull, touch, and feel everything within his. If you're just pregnant now, the hanging cords aren't an immediate threat, but trust us when we say that they *will* become irresistable to your baby.

According to Kevin . . .

I don't know what it is about those window cords with the plastic dangly ends, but babies and toddlers love to pull on them and the scary truth is that they are both a choking and a strangling hazard. Don't think on this too long. Just do something about it. Cut off, tie up, or use safety tassels on any dangling cords you have in the house now. Babies love to reach and grab—it's how they explore and expand their world. You want to give them the freedom to be able to do this without worry.

OK, so by now you're probably thinking, my baby is not even here yet and I'm already exhausted. Take a deep breath. You can't do it all at once, so focus on and feel good about what you can do, what you've *already* done. Also know that you just can't plan for everything—and what you have planned for is already making a difference.

According to Keith . . .

I put a lot of pressure on myself the first time around to make the nursery picture perfect. Nicole accused me of becoming a little obsessed. But, I was so proud that we had everything ready for Zachary's homecoming nearly a month before our due date. No one told us (or if they did we didn't listen) that when you first bring your baby home *he often doesn't even sleep in his own crib*! Zach slept in a bassinet in our room while the nursery that we'd knocked ourselves out to prepare was unoccupied. So my advice to you is, if you're feeling similarly crazed, try and relax. If the nursery isn't done by the time your baby is born, the upside is that she probably won't be sleeping in there for a few months anyway. The downside: Your room isn't just yours anymore!

Baby's world starts at the front door

The reality is that your baby's world extends outside his nursery; your baby's world starts at the front door. Think about it: If you've taken the time to pull up the carpeting and lay down natural-fiber rugs, cover the walls with low-VOC paint and open the windows and ventilate your baby's nursery, but you haven't changed a thing in the rest of the house, how baby-safe, really, is your home environment? If your goal is to create a baby-safe space where freedom is the ultimate goal, then the larger the baby-safe space, the more freedom, right? If you follow our thinking here, then it makes sense to apply the same set of health and safety standards for the nursery throughout your entire house—starting at the front door. Even though this takes a bit more time and effort, we believe it's well worth it and we're here to help.

Nursery. Check. Let's move on! Next up, you'll clean up *your* crib, starting with the kitchen and taking a detailed inventory of what you should keep and what you should throw out.

Step 1: Mommy Detox

Smart Solutions at a Glance

Glow Naturally

- Become familiar with the ingredients in your cosmetic and skincare products.
- Choose products that are primarily mineral-, plant-, and water-based.
- Switch to phthalate and fragrance-free skincare products

Arooma Therapy

- Crack your windows for a few minutes each day.
- Maintain your heating and air-conditioning units yearly.

- Consider installing ceiling fans to maximize ventilation and indoor airflow.
- Ditch manufactured synthetic fragrances and scents and opt for the smell of fresh, clean air.

A Tall Glass of (Clean) Water

- Run cold tap water every morning for a minimum of thirty seconds to flush out the pipes.
- Use cold water for drinking, preparing food, and mixing formula bottles.
- Unscrew your sink faucet aerators and clean the screens on a regular basis.
- Consider investing in a water filtration system.

A Healthy Plate for Two

- Eat produce lowest in pesticide residue or buy organic.
- Wash and lightly scrub all fruits and veggies with cold water before eating.
- Eat seafood with the lowest levels of mercury and limit yourself to two servings a week.

- Steer clear of unpasteurized milk and unpasteurized cheese.
- Cook all meat, poultry, and fish thoroughly and reheat leftovers well.

Decorate with Love

- Use low- or no-VOC paint.
- If you live in a home built prior to 1978, consider testing for lead.
- Replace old wall-to-wall carpeting with hardwood, bamboo, cork, or natural linoleum, or cover carpeting with easily washable, natural-fiber area rugs.
- Invest in a crib mattress or mattress pad and a changing-table pad filled with natural materials, like organic cotton or wool.
- Avoid build-your-own furniture made from pressed wood, plywood, and particleboard.
- Create a set of "healthy" and "safe" standards that can be applied throughout your entire living space.

Step 2

Crib Improvement

Pregnancy is the perfect time to take a good hard look at your products and habits with an eye to reducing exposure and potential harm. But you can start taking steps at *any time* to create a baby-safe environment for your whole family. After all, if it's baby-safe, it's family-safe, right?

In Step 1, you cleaned up your baby's nursery, but now . . . well, it's time to roll up your sleeves and *really clean* the rest of your crib. You'll begin by peering under your sinks, in your cabinets, the storage room, and garage and identifying anything and everything that could be tox-*ick*. We'll help you take it from there by sharing what we've learned about

- Safely purging harmful chemicals from your home
- Keeping a grime-free kitchen
- Why antibacterial products aren't always safe
- The down and dirty on floors
- How to rid your bathroom of mildew without toxins
- The secret to really "clean" laundry

After nearly a decade in the business of making natural, nontoxic cleaning products that are safe to use around babies, here's what we know: Most people don't think twice about the everyday household cleaners they use in their homes. And before starting babyganics we *were* those people. But we also know that more and more folks (like you!) are starting to think twice. Maybe you've given quite a bit of thought to the health and safety of the products you use to clean your home, or maybe you're just starting to wonder. What we've learned from talking to parents who are shopping in the baby-care aisles all over the country is that most families are cleaning their homes with the same cleaners they watched their parents use: "Hey, they worked for us. And we're all still alive!"

That may be true. But . . .

Most household cleaning products work at the expense of our health and safety, especially of the most vulnerable among us: our babies. This is an absolute fact. The research and information that proves this is available now where even twenty years ago it wasn't. Our parents and their parents sprayed and scrubbed with very little worry about safety because they didn't know, for example, that within twenty-six seconds of exposure to chemicals in many conventional household cleaning products, traces of those chemicals can be found in every organ in the body. Yeah. It turns out that what you don't know *can* hurt you.

The truth is that our parents and grandparents have likely been exposed to a bunch of nasty chemicals during their lifetimes. A lot of these chemicals have since been banned or removed from popular products, but just as quickly as old chemicals are taken off the shelves, new ones are being introduced. Today, there are over eighty-five thousand industrial chemicals in commercial production and many of them have not been tested, registered, or proven safe before they are put to use (you can blame the outdated Toxic Substances Control Act for that). On average, three new synthetics enter the market each day—chemicals that can be toxic, reactive, corrosive, even flammable! Not only that, but some of the "green," "all natural," and "earth-friendly" products, while pretty good at cleaning, contain harsh chemicals that pose significant risks to both the people who use them and everyone else in the house who comes into contact with them—especially, your baby.

Women and babies first

While the world has changed since our mothers and grandmothers scrubbed the tub, women still spend more time than men doing housework. Women spend *less* time cleaning now that working moms have become the norm in most households and the number of stay-at-home dads is twice that what it was ten years ago, and still, women do the bulk of the housework. As two guys who really do like to take a scouring pad to the floor (we're clean freaks!), we aren't happy about this stat. But it remains true. Women are regularly exposed to many more harsh chemicals and toxins. Just think about the cumulative impact of breathing, ingesting, and absorbing toxic chemicals on a regular basis. Many of these chemicals are absorbed readily into the body and have been linked to estrogenic cancers. Also consider that the very floors and surfaces that Mom regularly scrubs and wipes clean are where our babies and small children like to play, crawl, and snack. (If you spent the majority of your day this low to the ground, you'd probably eat off it, too.) Given their low-lying nature, our children are also at a higher risk of breathing, ingesting, and absorbing harmful contaminants found in many household cleaners.

Chemical Purge

You can pretty much assume that whatever you're using to clean your living space—your floors, tub, and countertops—is coming into direct and indirect contact with your little ones—both your babies and your pets. And if the ingredients in those cleaners have what's called a "high toxicity profile," they really are at risk. No need to panic, though. You're going to take a cool, calm, and methodical approach to cleaning house with small steps that, day after day, will eventually create a safer home for your family. Like we said earlier, our goal is to always make it safe, then let 'em play (rather than picking them up off the floor because it's dangerous).

Just as you did with your skincare products, you can easily begin to create a healthier home environment by simply becoming aware of which cleaners in your home might cause health issues and replacing them with products that are cleaner and safer. We're talking about a chemical purge, and it isn't just something we're into. After talking to so many of our customers, we've found that the "purge" or "cleanse" is sort of a ritual of new parenthood, kind of like the opposite of a traditional baby shower. Instead of acquiring new things for your baby, you're getting rid of stuff that's bad for them!

Come clean

When you take an inventory of the cleaning supplies you have stashed under your sinks, in your cabinets, and around your house, what do you find? Anything unnaturally blue? What do you smell? *Pee-yoo!* Is it strong? Does it smell fake? If you pop the top or use the product and the smell just isn't natural, chances are it's not! A lot of women tell us that when they were pregnant, their go-to household cleaners made them feel nauseated and dizzy. One woman, just a few months into her pregnancy, described not being able to smell or taste anything for two days after bleaching her bathroom tub. Not only is that unnatural—that's just not right! If a cleaning solution is hitting you that hard, imagine how it's affecting your baby.

We understand that product loyalty can run deep, especially when a product is tied to childhood memories. We've talked with a lot of parents who recall that as kids they associated a clean house with the residual headache they got from inhaling the artificial pine scent. For both of us, the smell of Clorox meant our high school locker room had just been de-grimed. But as we said earlier, in addition to being potentially harmful, a clean scent doesn't mean your home, office, or school is actually clean (or safe!).

Kevin and Keith's DOWNRIGHT-DIRTY List

CHLORINE BLEACH

Where you'll find it: Chlorine bleach, also known as sodium hypochlorite, has long been used as a disinfecting chemical. It's used to treat drinking water, sanitize swimming pools, and whiten laundry, including the sheets that go in your baby's crib. It's also commonly found in dishwasher detergents and bathroom and kitchen cleaners.

Why it's bad news: While chlorine bleach works to break down bacteria and other germs, it's registered by the EPA as a pesticide. At room temperature, chlorine becomes a highly corrosive gas that's a potent eye, skin, and respiratory irritant. If you've opened a bottle of bleach, you've experienced that *whoa* intense reaction to its fumes. Children are at an increased risk of exposure because they breathe twice as much air and at a much faster rate than adults, and are also more vulnerable to corrosive toxins because of the small diameter of their airways. When chlorine reacts with other elements, it can form disinfection by-products that may be damaging to human and embryonic tissue. The higher the concentration of the bleach, the more damage it can cause. Gloves and eye protection, as well as good ventilation, are commonly recommended for bleach use. We recommend not using it at all!

AMMONIA

Where you'll find it: Household cleaning solutions, specifically glass cleaners and multi-surface cleaners.

Why it's bad news: At room temperature, ammonia is a pungent, highly irritating gas and even exposure from inhalation to small amounts can cause burning of the eyes, nose, and throat. Choking and burning can occur with higher dosages. Did you know that when chlorine bleach and ammonia are mixed together, they create chloramine gas? We're talking about a chemical weapon used to poison people in World War I! Chloramine gas can cause bloody noses, neurological disorders, headaches, and even death. If you're housing either one of these dangerous agents, we suggest you come clean and throw them out.

TRICLOSAN AND TRICLOCARBON

Where you'll find them: Liquid dish and hand soaps, toothpaste, face wash, and deodorant; it's the active ingredient in most products labeled antibacterial and antimicrobial.

Why they're bad news: Triclosan and triclocarbon not only kill bacteria but may also mess with our human cells. They've been associated with low levels of thyroid hormone function, and may interfere with the body's production of estrogen and testosterone, which makes them leading suspects in causing breast and prostate cancer. One study detected triclosan and triclocarbon in the breast milk of mothers who use antibacterial products. Scientists are concerned that these antibacterial chemicals may also promote the growth of drug-resistant bacteria called superbugs.

SODIUM HYDROXIDE

Where you'll find it: Also known as lye and caustic soda, sodium hydroxide is a very strong chemical found in many household cleaning products such as oven cleaners and tub and tile cleaners, as well as in floor-stripping products, brick cleaners, and cements.

Why it's bad news: When inhaled, sodium hydroxide can create lung inflammation, sneezing, and throat pain and swelling. It can also cause burning of the nose, eyes, ears, lips, and tongue. If ingested, it can cause diarrhea, abdominal pain, and vomiting.

SOLVENTS

Where you'll find them: Cleaning and grease-cutting household products like stain removers, tub and tile cleaners, and toilet cleaners. Also found in laundry detergent, floor polish, rug cleaners, and oven cleaners.

Why they're bad news: When inhaled or touched, solvents can be very irritating to the skin, eyes, nose, and throat. Short-term exposure can cause dizziness or nausea. Potential longer-term exposure can cause birth defects, liver damage, and cancer.

SULFATES

Where you'll find them: Found in many laundry and dish detergents and in skincare products like shampoos, bubble bath, toothpaste, and body gels.

Why they're bad news: Sodium laureth sulfate (SLES) and its chemical cousin sodium lauryl sulfate (SLS) are the foaming agents in nearly every sudsy product in your house. SLS and SLES are considered safe by the FDA, while other health and environmental organizations classify them as "moderate hazards" that can be harsh and irritating to the skin. Since we believe all ingredients are guilty until proven innocent, we prefer to leave this class of sulfates out of our products. What's the harm in taking the safest approach?

ALCOHOL

Where you'll find it: hair spray, mouthwash, deodorant, perfume, aerosol surface cleaners, floor and furniture polish, and hand sanitizers.

Why it's bad news: Exposure can cause irritation of the eyes, nose, mouth, and throat. Repeated skin exposure can cause itching, rashes, and drying and cracking.

If your household cleaners make you feel itchy, rashy, dizzy, or sick, what are you waiting for? Purge them! Ditto if you know they contain any of the "downright dirty" ingredients above. They really are bad news for you and your baby.

Having said that, there's just one little problem: You probably won't know if the ingredients listed above are in your cleaning supplies; like it is with fragrance formulas, due to current "trade-secret" labeling laws there are no federal regulations requiring manufacturers of household products to list their ingredients. Whole Foods requires it but it's not a regulation. Some manufacturers post ingredients on their websites, but they're not required to. The truth is that makers of household cleaners can disclose whatever they want. Doesn't seem fair, does it? According to the National Research Council (an organization that seeks to improve government decision-making and public policy pertaining to science, engineering, and medicine), information about potentially toxic ingredients is unavailable for more than 80 percent of the chemicals in everyday-use products, including household cleaners, and many of those chemicals are harmful to you and your baby.

So how will you know what's in a product you are using and if it's actually safe? You probably won't, but what you *can* do is look for products that claim *not* to have the toxic ingredients listed earlier. Look for products with labels that say "no alcohol, phthalates, solvents and sulfates," for example. Also, read caution statements and warning labels carefully. While makers of household cleaners don't have to comprehensively list ingredients, if a known-to-be hazardous and harmful chemical is in the solution (carcinogens and reproductive toxicants fall into this category), a warning label *must* be visible on the bottle or package somewhere. So when you're taking an inventory of your household cleaners to decide on the safest choices for your family, look for "poison," "danger," "warning," and "caution" labels (much easier than scanning an ingredient list for unpronounceable chemicals, anyway). If

Helpful Resource: The NRDC's Label Lookup

When you're on the go (which as parents we so often are), with only a handful of minutes to get in and out of a store, the Natural Resources Defense Council's Label Lookup (iPhone app) can help you quickly make smart, safe, and informed product decisions. What does the label mean? Can you trust it? They've researched roughly 200 different claims that can be found on product labels so you don't have to! You can also access information about household products and their ingredients at the National Institutes of Health (NIH) household products database at householdproducts.nlm.nih.gov. If you want to take it a step further, contact the manufacturers of the products you buy to ask what *exactly* is in them. If any chemicals of concern are on the list, let them know you won't be buying their product until they find safer alternatives.

you come across a statement like "don't inhale or use in an unventilated area," or "dangerous to animals and humans," consider it *your warning not to use it*! Think about it, if you're using a tub and tile cleaner in your (likely) unventilated bathroom, how do you *not* inhale it? It's nearly impossible, which means the product is not safe. Permission to purge!

Q: Dear Founding Fathers,

I separated my cleaning supplies into two piles—the ones I want to get rid of and the ones I want to keep. What next? What do I do with all my open bottles of "toxic" cleaning supplies? How do I responsibly dispose of them?

A: Dear Dutiful Disposer,

You said the magic words: responsibly dispose. If you're about to pour the remains of a bottle down your sink or throw it out with the trash, stop right where you are. This is a big environmental no-no. The most responsible way to get rid of household cleaners containing potentially harmful or toxic ingredients is to take them to a hazardous waste facility where they can be disposed of safely. A little inconvenient, we know, but would you believe that about one percent of the nation's trash is made up of household hazardous waste? This may sound like a small amount, but it adds up to 3.36 million tons—an average of 60 to 100 pounds per household at any given time, some of which is probably within arm's reach of your children and pets, and considered so dangerous and toxic that to be safely disposed it should be handled by someone wearing a Hazmat suit.

According to Keith . . .

I'm like most guys in that I tend to, um, store a few things (OK, maybe *a lot of things*) in my garage. For a while, I had a ton of paint cans left over from home improvement projects I'd done over the years and that I'd kept around for touch-ups. Even though the paint had low or no VOCs, I knew storing that stuff long term was not a good idea. Even though I'd resealed all my cans good and tight, I understood that paint remnants can still become airborne and affect the quality of air in the house. Plus, paint is best stored in a cool, dry place and my garage is anything but in the hot and humid summer months. So one day, in a moment of sanity (and after a "healthy discussion" with my wife), I stacked them all in the back of the family car and drove them over to my nearest waste management facility (you can find where your local waste facility is by searching online). Mine wasn't exactly on my way to work, but it was the right thing to do, and it was a relief to get them off my hands. Since then, I've created a home improvement spreadsheet, listing what paints have been used on every wall in the

Helpful Resource: Handling Emergencies

Some parents really get into the "purge," disposing of everything toxic at once, where other parents prefer a steady-as-you-go approach, replacing one thing at a time. However you want to clean up your crib, it's cool with us, as long as you know exactly what to do if your child or pet comes into contact with something potentially toxic or hazardous in your home. Post the number for the American Association of Poison Control Centers' national emergency hotline, (800) 222-1222, in key locations throughout your home. Consider loading the American Red Cross's First Aid app to your smartphone, along with the Pocket First Aid and CPR app by the American Heart Association. If you haven't already, enroll in a CPR class led by a certified instructor (only takes an hour!), and always know the location of your nearest emergency room with pediatric expertise.

house, including the color and brand. Yeah, it's a little OCD, but it completely eliminates my excuse to keep old cans around for reference. More importantly, it's safer. If you're feeling reluctant to part with the cleaning supplies you've grown to love (one woman at a trade show admitted she'd cried after throwing out her old reliable tub and tile cleaner), remind yourself that this is about making safer choices for your family. Your mother and grandmother would be proud!

Clean with a clear conscience

OK, you've become aware of what you're using to scrub and scour and you've taken steps to purge your home of toxic troublemakers, all those bottles filled with blue unnatural stuff, but you still have to clean your home! What cleaning products will do the job and also allow your baby the freedom to safely explore her world?

As you might guess, we have a few ideas.

Fighting Grime

When we talk about cleaning solutions that are healthy and safe, we like to start at the kitchen sink because it's the gateway to your child's body. Think about it: The kitchen is where you wash and store everything that goes into your baby or child's mouth—bottles, pacifiers, teethers, sippy cups, plates, spoons, and forks, and if you're still using them, all those breast pump gadgets. Especially in the early weeks after your child is born, it's extra important to keep your kitchen clean and as free of toxic elements as possible. Things like chemical and gel residue from dish soaps can (and will!) find their way into your newborn's mouth, causing digestive discomfort and—worst-case scenario—leading to accidental poisoning.

According to Keith . . .

When Zach was born, it seemed like Nicole and I spent all of our "free time" (i.e. when Zack was napping) washing bottles and pacifiers. At the time, we were still using some traditional dish soap . . . you know, the kind that no matter how many times you rinse, still leaves a film? I remember thinking, "What the heck is in this stuff?" The residue that I had accepted as unavoidable was suddenly just not OK. I realized that if I couldn't get the dish soap off my hands, it must still be in the bottle and getting into my baby's mouth. How could that be safe? What we discovered when developing our babyganics foaming dish and bottle soap is that you can have it both ways: a product that's safe—free of alcohol, solvents, sulfates, phthalates, and fragrance—and effective at the same time.

Try It! babyganics Household Cleaners

There are many natural, nontoxic cleaning solutions out there, and as you know, we've developed a few of our own. Recommending our babyganics products might sound self-serving, but hey . . . we've spent a lot of time and energy working with an expert team of toxicologists, pediatricians, allergists, and researchers and developers to get our formulas just right. They're safe for you, your baby, your pets, and the environment. And, they're effective! We think they're pretty awesome (yeah, we're proud company daddies) and if you haven't already, consider checking them out. We promise: After you use them, your taste buds will still work!

Once you become more careful about what you use to wash your baby's, your family's, or dinner-party dishes (remember parties?) and switch to nontoxic soaps and cleaners, it's time to think about the tools you use to clean your house. Keep in mind that dishcloths, scrub brushes, and sponges can be a breeding ground for bacteria and a home for chemical contaminants and residue, along with your basic grime and gunk. How do you fight it? Wash your dishcloths and scrub brushes regularly in hot water, and clean your sponges by tossing them into the dishwasher or microwave, or by boiling them in water on the stove (warning: While it is effective, boiling dirty sponges does not produce a clean, fresh scent). We also recommend replacing your dishcloths, scrub brushes, and sponges regularly. Finally (and this really goes without saying), dry clean dishes, utensils, surfaces, and your hands with a freshly laundered dish towel.

Q: **Dear Founding Fathers,**

How careful do I have to be about my baby's bottles? I'm still breast-feeding. Should I wash them with antibacterial soap?

A: **Dear Bottle Wary,**

Great question! When it comes to using an antibacterial substance on your baby's bottles or anything your baby could come into contact with, we're pretty insistent—don't! Use a natural soap and water instead. Get this: In 2005 the FDA found no proof that antibacterial soaps are in any way superior to soap and water in preventing the spread of germs. The truth is that simple soap and water is *just as effective* and *much safer*. You see, antibacterial substances were not created with your baby in mind. In fact, most weren't created with the *planet* in mind. The majority of antimicrobial soaps on the market today contain triclosan, a chemical that when mixed with water and sunlight—both readily available at your kitchen sink—can become a toxic dioxin. Even low levels of dioxins are harmful. These environmental pollutants have been linked to reproductive and developmental problems, especially in women and young children, and may also mess with the immune system, interfere with hormones, and cause cancer. No thanks! We strongly recommend that you pass on this stuff. If you've been using it up to now, don't freak. It's OK. Just make the switch. We all worry about germs. It's hard to imagine that getting rid of them can do more harm than good. Now you know.

A Safe Germinator

This is going to go against everything you've been told in advertising—the best way to kill germs and eliminate bacteria from our homes is to use antibacterial hand soap, cleaners, sprays, and wipes—but the truth is antibacterial products actually do more harm than good. This is why we're anti-antibacterial. Not only can they create toxic dioxins, but the overuse of "germ-killing," "antimicrobial" products creates stronger bacteria and resistant viruses called superbugs that our babies' bodies have a harder time fighting off. Many experts we talked to also theorize that overusing antibacterial products that lower our body's resistance makes allergies and asthma in our children more likely.

Another good reason to stay away from antibacterial products is that one of the key ingredients is alcohol, which can be very drying and irritating to a baby's sensitive skin, and can hurt, burn, and sting when used on scrapes, scratches, and cuts or eczema-prone face and hands . . . Ouch!

Alcohol is easily absorbed into the skin, but it's even more dangerous to *ingest* antibacterial products. Would you believe that most alcohol-based sanitizers contain 62 percent alcohol? Some contain 70 percent! That's more than vodka! Drinking some of that can make a baby or child very nauseated and sick, and drinking a lot could be fatal.

According to Kevin . . .

Over the holidays, my son Tyler came home with a gift from his teacher—a small bottle of hand sanitizer with an alcohol content of 60+ percent and a picture of a sugar cookie on the label. I popped the top and took a whiff and sure enough, the sanitizer had a "cookie dough" scent. It smelled delicious. I imagined his bus ride home—a bunch of five-year-olds without much adult supervision and no one to warn, "Hey, kids, I know this may smell like a bottle of yummy liquid cookies, but please don't drink it because it might actually kill you!"

In 2011, the American Association of Poison Control Centers got 13,974 reports of children under age five swallowing antibacterial sanitizers. One of them, a five-year-old girl from Michigan, had sampled a chocolate-and-strawberry-scented sanitizer and was later rushed to the hospital after vomiting and losing consciousness! This is the result of misleading and very harmful messaging. Like a lot of products, antibacterial hand sanitizers are heavily marketed to our kids, so much so that teen abuse of alcohol-based hand sanitizer (yeah, abuse by drinking it) is on the rise. At one college, students discovered that not only did drinking antibacterial hand soap give them a buzz, it was also flammable. So . . . they lit shots of it on fire, *and then drank it*! And these kids got into college! As far as we're concerned these products have no place on a college campus, in schools for our young children, or in a home with babies. Period.

As parents, one of our biggest pet peeves is that we have little control over what our children are exposed to when they're away from home, whether at day care, summer camp, school, or even playdates and birthday parties. But instead of being annoying helicopter parents who bring their own products wherever they go (um . . . we've been those guys), we try to focus on educating and empowering parents like you with the knowledge we've gained over the years so that you can make safer choices for your family, too.

According to Keith . . .

My son Zach's first big birthday party was at one of those bouncy-gym places. We were all excited, but when my wife and I got there we saw alcohol-based hand sanitizer dispensers on nearly every wall in the place. Then we saw the bright blue cleaning solution the employees were spraying all over the toys that Zach and his friends were about to touch, climb on, and, no doubt, lick. *Uh-oh.* We'd been so wrapped up in making Zach's party perfect that we'd overlooked some obvious safety concerns that we should have taken into account. Big teachable moment here—learn as much as you can about the environment you're exposing your child to and then decide what you're comfortable with. Had we known we'd be walking into a space sprayed down with bleach and toxic ammonia, we might have chosen somewhere else to celebrate.

Don't buy the "antimicrobial" hype

Given all these safety concerns, why is the use of these products so widespread? Why is "antibacterial" and "antimicrobial" slapped on nearly every label out there, and how did we all become convinced we needed to eliminate bacteria from our homes? The short answer is: marketing. The longer answer is: There are some situations where antibacterial products serve an important purpose, just not in everyday life.

Antibacterial products were developed for use in hospitals and clinical settings. They help to maintain a sterile environment so people who are sick and have compromised immune systems are protected from potentially life-threatening germs, especially where there's a heightened risk of introducing new infection during invasive procedures like surgery. In clinical settings like these, disinfecting is absolutely critical to the health of many patients—the benefits outweigh the risks. So yes, there is a place for antibacterial products. But your home is probably not it. You can achieve an effective level of cleanliness without treating your kitchen like it's an operating room. Antibacterial products are good for surgeons, not so good for parents. In your world, they're just not necessary.

Q: Dear Founding Fathers,
What if someone sick comes to my home and is around my baby? Wouldn't this be the right time to use germ-killing, antibacterial products?

A: Dear Safe or Sorry,
Unless that someone sick lives in your home, our suggestion is that you keep the sickness at bay, and by that we mean—*away*. Keep the sick person out of the house and away from your baby. Sure, you might offend a friend or family member who wants to visit your newborn, but if they show up with a cold, you might gently suggest they come back when they are feeling better. Lathering up with an antibacterial soap before cuddling your baby doesn't mean germs won't spread. Also, an alcohol-based sanitizer isn't something that should come into contact with your new baby's sensitive and easily irritable skin.

The way we see it, one of the benefits and responsibilities of becoming a parent is that it gives you a new opportunity to redefine the standards of what's healthy and safe for your family. Remember—you're the parent. You get to make your own house rules!

That's our general take on antibacterial products, so let's wash our hands (in ole reliable soap and water) of this debate for now, and finish cleaning house.

Floors to Adore

You've tackled the kitchen. Now, it's time to look down toward your feet. Yeah, we covered the floors in Step 1, but we think they're worth another once-over because keeping this hand-to-mouth, down-and-dirty crawling zone clean is super critical to your baby's health.

Remember, your baby's room starts at the front door and eight-five percent of the gunk we bring into the home comes in on the bottom of our shoes and on our pets' paws. Allergy- and asthma-producing dust, pet dander, bacteria, mildew, mold, and chemical residue that compromise our indoor air quality is brought in by our feet, heightening our babies' exposure to a lot of potentially harmful stuff. So kick off your shoes as soon as you walk in the front door. This practice isn't just about being polite. It's one of the safest things you can do!

Clean gently from top to bottom

To a home with kids, floors are a place to play, sleep, crawl, eat, roll around, and learn to walk. They're no place for cleaners that contain harsh chemicals, so again, when cleaning your home, we suggest using plant-based cleaning solutions with no alcohol, parabens, sulfates, phthalates, or toxins. When it comes to cleaning your hardwood, bamboo, cork, or natural linoleum floors, we also suggest that rather than dry sweeping, you use a damp mop with a sponge or a string-type mop head, or spot clean with a damp cloth. This limits the amount of surface dust, dirt, and dander you might kick up into the air during the cleaning process. Finally, when cleaning carpets and rugs, avoid shaking and beating. Wet scrub or spot clean with a damp cloth. Now, your little ones are ready for action!

Your floors are the largest surface in your home, yet it's just as important to keep *all* your surfaces clean. Truth is, when our countertops, coffee tables, and blinds aren't clean, our floors aren't either, because any dirt, dust, and grime that's collected above will eventually travel through the air and drift down to the floor. So, clean from high to low and you're good to go. Really, there's no point making your floors shine if you aren't also giving everything above them the same love and attention.

When cleaning surfaces, we suggest using soft, dampened, and disposable cloths or rags rather than steel wool, scouring pads, and abrasive cleaners, which can easily generate more dust and airborne allergens. While paper towels fall into the disposable cloth category, unless you use unbleached, recyclable paper towels, we suggest leaving them off your next grocery list. Our reasons: Paper towels are not great for the environment, they're expensive, and you can conveniently clean and pick up spills with materials you already have lying around the house. To clean up messes, we like to use old cotton T-shirts and cloth diapers. Smart, huh? Another way to go is investing in a chemical-free microfiber cloth, which can substitute for over sixty rolls of paper towels before it needs replacing. Handy!

Scrub-a-Tub-Tub

It looks innocent enough, but the scrub-a-tub-tub is where you and your family are at your most vulnerable. By which we mean . . . naked. Not where you want to greet scum and mildew or chemical residue from cleaning products. Besides just being gross, bacteria, mold, and mildew can trigger asthma and allergies, and sometimes make you feel like you've got the flu! They thrive in moist places, so cleaning the bathroom regularly is a must. But you need to be careful. Traditional tub, toilet, and tile cleaners are some of the biggest (if not *the biggest*) toxic offenders on the market. When their fumes build up in small, unventilated places, watch out skin, eyes, and throat! Many of the "natural," "eco-friendly," and "green" cleaners out there are less than benign, too. While a natural tub and tile cleaner is likely made of ingredients that don't pose the same environmental dangers as a traditional cleaner, they can be harmful to you and your baby if inhaled or ingested.

According to Keith . . .

Nicole and I had a "moment" the first time we put Zach in the tub. He was so small, and his skin was so soft and delicate. When we turned on the water, we were hit with the awareness that whatever we were using to clean the tub was coming into direct contact with his precious skin. It was like—OMG, what's touching our baby? And, is it safe? Once we did our homework and learned that many of the chemicals in traditional household tub and tile cleaners have been linked to reproductive and hormone disruption, allergies, asthma, and even psychological disorders like ADHD, we said, "That's it!" We purged any remaining traditional cleaners we had in the house and replaced them with natural, nontoxic formulas.

Keep your bathroom dry and moisture free and you'll minimize the growth and spread of bacteria, which means you'll spend less time on your hands and knees scrubbing your toilet and tub. This will allow you time to do something else—like take a hot shower—by yourself! In addition, try the following smart solutions to keep mold and mildew to a minimum.

SMART SOLUTIONS:
Hold the Mold

- Pop a window. Our bathrooms tend to be hot spots for heavy, humid, and unventilated air, so open a window to release trapped air.
- Ventilate. Improve the air quality in your bathroom by flipping on the fan while you shower and bathe. Once you've toweled off, leave the door standing open.

- Dry off. Get into the habit of wiping down the surfaces of your tub and counters when moist.
- Dehumidify. Improve the soggy air quality in your bathroom; use a dehumidifier to soak up moisture.

Adopting these smart solutions will really help to minimize the growth of bacteria in your bathrooms, but the slimy grime has a mind of its own. Despite your best efforts, mildew and mold will find a way to sneak in. In these cases, we suggest facing it head-on with a natural, nontoxic cleaner that really works (our babyganics Tub and Tile Cleaner contains no parabens, sulfates, or phthalates) but leaves no harmful residue behind.

Q: **Dear Founding Fathers,**

I'm looking for alternatives to over-the-counter cleaners—something I can make myself with simple and natural ingredients that I might already have at home. What do you recommend?

A: **Dear Do-It-Yourselfer,**

Hey, we're born do-it-yourselfers! So we're happy to provide you with a few of our favorite DIY grime-fighter solutions.

Vinegar: Also known as acetic acid, distilled white vinegar has been used for ages on glass and windows because it produces a clean, streak-free shine. (Shhh: It's the secret weapon for removing watermarks on drinking glasses.) Because it's highly acidic, vinegar also works wonders to destroy bacteria, mold, and soap scum. What's more, you can find it most anywhere, and it's dirt cheap.

Essential oils: Essential oils like thyme, rosemary, clove, eucalyptus, and oregano have natural antibacterial properties and add a nice fragrance to your DIY "green" cleaners. Many essential oils also work as effective bug repellents. For example, wiping down your cabinets and countertops with rosemary oil helps keep household roaches away from the kitchen.

Baking soda: No matter how much you clean, sometimes you can't get rid of that funky smell. Try leaving an open box of baking soda under your sinks (always out of reach of children) to neutralize and absorb stinky odors.

Castille soap: In most circumstances, simple soap and water attacks grit and grime just as well as any other cleanser.

Take a Load Off

Just as important as cleaning your dishes, surfaces, furniture, and floors with safe, nontoxic products is switching to a laundry detergent that is free of synthetic fragrances and dyes, and tossing out any and all laundry detergents, stain removers, and fabric softeners that contain harsh chemicals.

We've met a lot of parents who have embraced the importance of washing their baby's clothes, blankets, and bibs with gentle ingredients, but they don't do the same for themselves. If you separate your laundry into grown-up and baby piles, consider consolidating into one basket. You deserve the same safety and comfort as your baby, don't you? The answer is yes! Plus, think of how often your baby snuggles up against you. When your clothes have been washed with laundry detergents that contain harsh chemicals and synthetic fragrances, guess whose button nose is getting a strong whiff of them? Many laundry detergents, stain removers, and fabric softeners can trigger allergies and irritate our babies' skin, and if you're a breast-feeding mama, smelling synthetically "baby fresh" could also become a problem. Did you know that some breast-fed babies won't latch on and nurse if Mom smells suspiciously . . . *not like Mom?* Makes you rethink what it means to do a load of "clean" laundry, doesn't it?

In addition to switching to laundry detergents, stain removers, and fabric softeners that are safer for you and your baby, try extending that same consideration to the world your little ones will inherit.

SMART SOLUTIONS:

Come Clean!

- Maximize. Small loads of laundry waste water and energy, so wait until you've got a full load before doing one (and with babies and kids in the house, that doesn't take long). Washing only full loads of laundry at the proper water level setting (see our next tip) will ensure that each load is using the optimal amount of energy.
- Turn down the heat. Did you know that by washing the bulk of your

laundry in cold water, you could save big in energy costs every month? Even changing from hot to warm water will save you some money. According to the Department of Energy, switching from hot to warm water can cut your energy costs nearly in half! When drying clothes, choose a cooler setting as well. (The exception to this "cool rule" is when washing new clothes to remove chemical residue left over from the manufacturing process and when washing bedding, where allergy-inducing dust mites like to hide out. Wash and dry these loads on HOT.)

- Air dry. Even on cool, your clothes dryer eats up a sizeable amount of energy. If you can, dry your clothes outside on a clothesline on breezy, warm days. Line drying uses no energy. If you don't have the outdoor space, make space in your laundry room for a drying rack.
- Wear it more than once. Aside from underwear and socks (duh!), our best recommendation for cutting back on your laundry is to just do less of it. By wearing your favorite jeans more than once before tossing them in the dirty pile, you can consume up to *five times less energy* on a regular basis. And when you wash them in cold water and hang them on a line to dry, you save even more energy and reduce your carbon footprint.

OK. Now that you've done a deep clean of your house, it's time to shift focus to adopting healthy habits and smart solutions for keeping your baby squeaky-clean, too! Next . . . washing your baby's body!

Smart Solutions at a Glance

Chemical Purge

- Create a healthier environment by becoming aware of which cleaners in your home might cause health issues and replace them with products that are cleaner and safer.
- Our general rule of thumb: If it's blue, get rid of it! Also, if the smell just isn't natural, chances are it's not!
- Be on the lookout for products with caution statements and warning labels, such as "poison," "danger," and "caution"—you may want to steer clear of them.

Fighting Grime

- Switch to natural, nontoxic cleaners that are free of alcohol, solvents, sulfates, phthalates, and fragrance.
- Wash your dishcloths and scrub brushes regularly in hot water, and clean your sponges by tossing them into the dishwasher or microwave, or by boiling them.

A Safe Germinator

- Avoid using alcohol-based antibacterial or antimicrobial soaps. Use natural soap and water instead.
- Learn as much as you can about the environment you're exposing your child to and then decide what you're comfortable with.

Floors to Adore

- Kick off your shoes as soon as you walk in the front door.
- Use plant-based cleaning solutions with no alcohol, parabens, sulfates, phthalates, or toxins to clean floors.
- Rather than dry sweeping, use a damp mop, cloth, or sponge to spot clean.

Scrub-a-Tub Tub

- Keep your bathroom dry and moisture-free and you'll minimize the growth and spread of bacteria and mold.
- Pop a window to release trapped air and ventilate your bathroom by flipping on the fan while you shower and bathe.

- Get into the habit of wiping down the surfaces of your tub and counters so moisture doesn't collect and create mold.

Take a Load Off

- Switch to a laundry detergent, stain remover, and fabric softener that are free of synthetic fragrances and dyes.
- If you separate your laundry into grown-up and baby piles, consider consolidating into one basket.
- Wash the bulk of your laundry in cold water and dry on a cooler setting, and you will reduce your carbon footprint and save money in energy costs.

Step 3

Baby Comforts

OK, home tour? Check! Purged toxic waste from your cabinets and shelves? Check! Now it's time to focus on the products that touch your baby: soap, shampoo, lotions, diapers, and wipes—anything and everything that come into direct contact with your baby's delicate and vulnerable skin.

Want to know just how delicate and vulnerable? How about this: Your baby's skin is five times thinner than yours. That's wafer thin! As you can imagine, skin that thin is highly sensitive—especially during the first full year of life—making it susceptible to moisture loss and more vulnerable to toxins, pollutants, and irritants. Since you're becoming more conscious of the health and safety of household products such as a tile cleaner that may indirectly come into contact with your child, now you really have to consider what's coming into *direct* contact—straight from the bottle or tube—with your baby's skin, from belly to cheeks (all four of them!). We'll introduce you to products that are safer for your baby's skin and share what we've learned about

- The importance of proper hand hygiene
- How to protect and soothe your baby's kissy face
- What makes for healthy, safe, and fun tub time
- Tending to your baby's tushy

Fine and Handy

Did you know that cold and flu germs can live on surfaces like door handles, grocery carts, high chairs, bathroom floors, and changing tables for days? Ewww! And other viruses can survive this way for months. Double Ewww! Which is why good hand washing is by far the best way for all of us to avoid the transfer of germs that can make your whole family sick. Honestly, if you can teach your children to do *just one thing* to prevent the spread of germs and infections, it's how to properly wash and clean hands. Teach this at an early age and you set your little ones up with a healthy habit for life. And believe it or not, you can begin teaching your baby this valuable lesson in the first few months of life.

As parents, we've both discovered something you've probably already learned yourself. Kids (even babies!) are brilliant mimics. They copy everything we do. So we figure to instill healthy practices and safe habits in our kids, we have to represent them in a way that makes sense and is also fun. The best part about hand hygiene is that washing hands is a simple solution that kids *get*; the idea that a) hands carry dirt and icky germs and b) clean hands are healthy makes plain sense to them. And, with just a little bit of forethought, you can make hand washing *fun*. Make up your own games and competitions at the sink—whose hands are cleaner or who washed their hands first? Wash your hands alongside them. Play little finger games. Before you know it, you've got a foamy giggle-fest on your hands. Just because it's important, doesn't mean it has to be serious!

According to Keith . . .

We always say if you want to create good, healthy family habits, you better start with yourself. Nicole and I are kind of nuts about hand washing, and when we first had kids we knew that we were going to raise little hand washers. We were determined to make hand washing high on our "fun family activities" list. So yeah, we came up with our own silly hand-washing song and sang it when we washed their hands and when we washed our own. (I've been known to sing it to myself at the sink in the office men's room. Just saying.) We also used the baby hand sign for "washing hands" every time we took the kids to the sink. We believe that repetition creates ritual, and at around ten months old, Zach proved us right when he pointed to the sink and made the sign for "wash." Nicole and I gave each other a high five for a job well done. (Then we washed our hands.)

From very early on, both of our older kids have washed their hands without giving us a hard time; that's because we made it playful. We'd splash around and make volcanoes out of foam. As our kids got older, more willful and independent, and their hand-washing enthusiasm started to wane, we introduced rewards. Both Zach and Skylar were given their own special hand towel (which they got to pick out), and after every good washing we'd reward them with at least a hug. Bigger prizes included stickers. Now it's become a healthy habit they don't even think about. Recently, I overheard Zach saying, "Wash your hands before snack," to one of his friends. That's my boy!

Lather, rinse, repeat

Most of us don't spend a lot of time thinking about the mechanics of hand washing. What's to think about? You turn on the water, wash your hands, and towel off, right? It's just that simple until you become a parent and all of sudden you're supposed to be the expert. As soon as we became dads, it occurred to us that we weren't 100 percent sure how to teach our kids proper hand-washing technique. Was there a "right" way, and if so—what was it? We had to relearn the basics, so we'll assume you need a refresher course, too. As long as you're washing, might as well do it right. Right? (Hey, even heart surgeons have to learn this stuff . . .)

Teach your children to follow these basic hand-washing steps: lather your hands with soap and warm water. Wash from top to bottom, front and back, scrubbing between your fingers as you go. Did you know that it's actually the friction and the length of time you wash and not the soap that's doing the majority of the germ killing? Rinse and repeat for thirty to sixty seconds, the equivalent of singing the ABC's twice. Dry off with a clean hand towel. Done.

Our kids really do learn by watching, so master your own hand-washing technique before you expect them to monkey see, monkey do. Also, become a more frequent hand-washer. Let your children see you wash your hands in a variety of everyday situations—after using household cleaners, before prepping food, after wiping a runny nose, before washing dishes—and they'll quickly learn that hand washing is just something you do without thinking much about it!

Q: Dear Founding Fathers,

Teaching my kids about hand washing was pretty easy. It's harder to teach the grown-ups who come through my front door! I even got into an argument with my dad about the importance of hand hygiene. He tried to tell me that unless you're sick, giving your hands a quick "rinse off" with water is enough to keep them clean. His reasoning: If you're healthy, your hands aren't dirty. *For real?* I admit that I've become more careful since bringing my newborn daughter home from the hospital, but running water over your hands is not good enough. Am I a clean freak or . . . just clean?

A: Dear Clean (but Not a Freak),

You're right that a new baby is more susceptible to viruses and bacteria, so it is a safe idea for anyone who could be sick to make sure their hands are good and clean before handling your baby (or better yet, as we mentioned earlier, keep their hands *off* your baby). And we're not trying to start a family feud here but, um, your dad is wrong. Rinsing off doesn't do much and you don't have to be sick to spread bacteria and germs, chemical residue, pet saliva, and whatever your hands come into contact with throughout the day. Don't forget you can feel perfectly healthy and still be infected with a cold or a flu that hasn't manifested yet. Did you know some viruses can live for up to eight hours outside the body? We're with you on this one; it's completely appropriate—and not rude—to ask everyone who comes into your home to wash their hands properly—that is, with soap and warm water—before touching your baby. Remember, it's your baby, your rules!

When dirty germs happen to clean people

Even if you wash your hands all the time, you can still get sick. That's just a fact of family life, of having babies and kids around the house. Sickness happens. From time to time our babies and toddlers are going to bump into a big bully of a germ and get knocked down. While doing research for this book and in speaking to our A-Team of doctors and researchers, we came across this crazy statistic—the average number of viral infections that a preschooler gets per year is eight. For kindergartners, it's twelve. Each lasts for seven to ten days and occurs between the months of October and April. When you add it all up, that's eighty to one hundred days of sickness over a six-month period. That's what we call a headache! But aside from the professional inconvenience that many sick days creates, along with the mountain of snot you're in charge of wiping up, a sick baby isn't necessarily a bad thing. Fighting germs is how our children build up their immune systems so that they can grow stronger.

Still, understanding that germs are a part of life doesn't mean your baby has to pick up every virus at the playground. To avoid sickness (or passing it on to someone else, like *you*!), your baby's best defense—hands down—is for us to adopt the following smart solutions at home and in public settings like at day care and the park, where germs thrive and multiply.

SMART SOLUTIONS:
Keep Germs Away!

- Sharing is good, but . . . learn *not* to share foods, drinks, or utensils.
- Wash hands after playing with other children's toys.
- Wash hands before meals and snacks.
- Avoid touching eyes, nose, and mouth (not so easy for little ones, so simply encourage them to try their best).
- Cover your cough like a Count (Dracula!)—into your elbow fold and not your hand.
- Blow that runny nose frequently.

Q: Dear Founding Fathers,

I just went back to work full time, so my eight-month-old is now in day care. She's thriving there socially and intellectually, but *I swear*, it's like she comes home with some kind of new virus every other week. What can I do to prevent her from picking up anything and everything out in the real world? Is it even possible to avoid germs in a day-care environment?

A: Dear Wannabe Germ-Free Mommy,

Keeping kids free of germs in the real world is not an easy job, and this is especially true in day-care facilities. You have to consider that like most eight-month-olds, your daughter probably has a natural predisposition (those grabby, touchy hands!) for carrying and spreading germs around. Not only might she pick up something from an object like a block or a book, but she's also in constant and close contact with lots of other kids. Germs are hard to avoid! Also consider that her day-care provider may not have received appropriate hygiene training for avoiding the spread of infection. Yup, the simple fact is that many day cares have extremely high employee turnover rates and are not always able to provide training on simple solutions, like proper hand hygiene. So when choosing a day care or preschool for your little one, do your research. You may first consider asking your pediatrician for his or her top picks for "germ-free" schools. As a caregiver for many children in your area, your pediatrician will have great insight on which facilities have the healthiest track records. Then, before you enroll your child in any one program, take a tour. Watch closely, listen, and learn. Are the following smart solutions being put into place? If not, you may want to cross that school off your list and continue your search.

SMART SOLUTIONS:

Clean and Healthy Day Care

- Frequent hand washing. Studies have shown that proper hand washing is the best way to limit the spread of infection and germs in day-care centers.
- Minimize sickness. While it's impossible to totally prevent the spread of germs in the day-care environment, watch to see that caregivers are teaching the children to cover their sneezes and coughs, and that runny noses are wiped immediately.
- Find small day-care groups. This limits the number of children who can spread icky germs.
- Alcohol-free hand soaps and nontoxic cleaners. Does the facility frequently clean surfaces using soaps and products made especially with your child's health and safety in mind? Remember, cleaners don't have to be toxic to work!
- Clean diapering stations and potties. Foot-activated trash cans for diapers is the best solution for reducing the transfer of infectious crud on hands. Use of disposable latex gloves and good sanitation of diapering areas are also important ways to prevent the spread of germs.
- Proper food preparation. Porous, cracked, or damaged plates and surfaces can provide bacteria safe havens to hide out. Look for facilities where the counters and dishware are in good condition and kept clean. Food prep should be done a good distance away from diaper-changing areas.

- Caregiver training. Do your homework. Have the caregivers been properly trained on hygiene practices for limiting the spread of infectious microbes?
- Look for a day care with an open-door policy, so you can pop in at any time and see what's going on.

Make healthy hands a habit

You've already heard our anti-antibacterial rant, but still, we know that breaking the hand-sanitizer habit can be as hard as taking a bottle from a baby. So we'll say it again: Lathering "germ-killing" soap on your baby's hands during flu and cold season isn't a bad call (after all, hands are little tide pools for nasty bacteria), but—and it's a BIG but!—alcohol-based, antibacterial hand soap and sanitizer is not only ineffective, it's also unhealthy and unsafe—on your child's dishes, cups, and bottles, and on her delicate face and hands. Think about it: When babies and children suck on their fingers and stick their hands in their mouths (as just about every child we've ever met does), they risk exposure to toxic residue these soaps leave behind. So even at the height of flu and cold season, stick to simple soap and water. It's skin-friendly and just as effective!

Q: **Dear Founding Fathers,**

What if I'm somewhere where I don't have access to soap and water?

A: Dear Soap-Stranded,

When it comes to your hands specifically, if basic hand washing isn't an option (you're at the park, stuck in the car, or the public bathroom line is just too darn *long*), hand sanitizing with an *alcohol-free* hand sanitizer is a good backup plan (but only a backup plan, OK?). If you're a parent who's regularly on the go, it's not a bad idea to have some stashed in your car, or your baby's stroller or diaper bag. (Try our babyganics alcohol-free, foaming hand-sanitizing spray and wipes.)

Kissy Face

Now that we've given you more than an earful about hands, go ahead and give them a rest. Let's move on to how best to protect your baby's kissy face from harmful outside influences—allergens, chemical irritants, and the blasted sun!

It's pretty obvious every time you kiss 'em that babies are not born with a tough skin. Their naturally thin and sensitive skin takes years to thicken up. This means hydrating and moisturizing from day one is an absolute must, and yet many of the baby skincare products on the market that claim to protect and soothe actually contain ingredients that do just the opposite! Additives like artificial dye and synthetic fragrances are just too tough for your sensitive baby's skin! They tend to dry out and irritate little lips, cheeks, and noses—neither gentle in the short term, nor safe over time.

Kevin and Keith's

TOO-TOUGH-FOR-THIN-SKIN List

ARTIFICIAL DYES

Where you'll find them: Personal care products for babies and grown-ups like bubble baths, bath soaps, and shampoos to either create a color or mask a color.

Why they're bad news: They're unnecessary and can irritate and provoke allergies.

MINERAL OIL

Where you'll find it: Also known as liquid petroleum, mineral oil is a key ingredient in many baby oils, lotions, diaper-rash creams, ointments, and lip balms.

Why it's bad news: Petrochemicals such as mineral oil form a layer on the skin and can seal pores and trap dirt and bacteria, making it hard for your baby's skin to eliminate sweat and toxins and heal, and also to absorb beneficial vitamins and minerals.

When creating products for our babyganics skincare line, we keep in mind that anything you put on your baby's skin is a potential irritant. Our philosophy is: Less is more. So we stay away from ingredients that could harm the skin, like sulfates and synthetic fragrances, and instead use plant-based ingredients, like colloidal oatmeal, comfrey, cucumber, and chamomile, and natural moisturizers like cocoa seed butter, shea butter, and avocado that are soothing and nourishing to a baby's developing skin. As protective fathers, we believe that these products should prepare our babies' skin for their first exposure to the world, as well as nurture and support their skin's development over the years. Would you agree? We kind of thought you would.

Q: **Dear Founding Fathers,**

My son has itchy, sensitive eczema-prone skin and I feel like I've tried everything to treat it. Nothing seems to work. Or if it does, it doesn't for long. Could the products I'm using be causing the eczema?

A: **Dear Irritated,**

That depends on what you're using. Dry, itchy eczema is an allergic reaction. It's often triggered by foods (peanuts, wheat, cow's milk, and eggs are common culprits) and everyday products like laundry detergents and bath soap, which can contain perfumes and artificial dyes that aggravate the skin. Because your baby's young and sensitive skin is five times thinner than yours, it's much more susceptible to moisture loss and more vulnerable to irritants, so if you're using a skincare product with harsh chemicals, it's very possible that the product could be the cause of, or at least significantly contributing to, your son's eczema flare-ups.

While your pediatrician is the best person to diagnose your son's eczema and determine the culprit, you can begin to treat your baby's itchy and rashy discomfort by considering the smart solutions below.

SMART SOLUTIONS:
Bye-Bye Dry

- Avoid the big triggers. Eczema is an allergic reaction, often to specific foods and/or environmental and household toxins. Check with your pediatrician to see if your child has a food allergy. If she does, you may need to avoid skincare products made with nuts, milk, and gluten. (Our products are labeled accordingly.) As a general rule, avoid skincare products with perfumes, synthetic dyes, and alcohol, all of which can dry out and irritate your baby's skin.
- Check irritants off your laundry list. If your child is suffering from red, itchy, or bumpy skin, consider what you're using to wash clothes and bedding. If you haven't yet made the switch to a natural, fragrance-free laundry detergent, now's the time! Using a natural detergent with no harsh chemicals will allow you to check "irritants" off your laundry list!
- Do another home tour. Your baby's nursery starts at the front door, so take another walk through your entire living space. Consider everything your baby's coming in contact with—bedding, carpeting, furniture, and

household cleaners, even the indoor air. If you pinpoint something that could be irritating your baby's skin, remove it and see what happens.

- Humidify. Eczema tends to flare up in the winter months when it's cold outside and dry inside, so consider investing in a humidifier to pump up the moisture level in your baby's nursery. Just be sure to regularly clean it and keep it dry between uses. Bacteria is drawn to water and a humidifier provides the perfect breeding ground.
- Bathe a little less. Frequent bathing can dry out your baby's skin, so consider saving the bath for only two or three times a week, and when you lather up, be sure to use a natural moisturizing soap and reduce the overall soak time. In other words, keep baths short and sweet; the less your baby sits in the water, the less her skin will dry out.
- Wash on the mild side. Skin dries out faster in hot water, so keep your baby's bathwater cool.
- Apply often. To treat itchy and scratchy eczema, apply the *three R*'s: rehydrate, replenish, repeat! Immediately after bath time apply a generous amount of cream or emollient to the red and inflamed dry areas to seal in moisture. Also, get into the habit of reapplying a moisturizing and protective cream throughout the day (after every diaper change), and especially in the winter months when cold climates tend to accelerate drying and chapping. The the *three R*'s will help seal in your baby's natural body moisture and create a protective barrier between her skin and external irritants.
- Dress lightly. Dress and swaddle your child in soft and cool natural fabrics, like cotton. There's nothing worse than itchy wool or heavy swad-

dling blankets when your skin is *already* itchy and dry. Think light and airy—let your baby's skin breathe and heal.

- Cut 'em short. What do we do when we have an itch? We scratch it! Unfortunately, when our babies seek relief this way, they often make the itch worse. Scratching and rubbing can further irritate or inflame eczema-prone skin, so keep those little fingernails short. And if he just can't keep his hands off himself, put him to bed in cotton mittens or socks.
- Cool it down. To soothe itchy, painful flare-ups, try applying cool compresses to the area, along with moisturizers throughout the day.
- Probiotics. Many parents swear by introducing flaxseed oil and probiotic, bacteria-friendly foods like kefir into their children's diets to help with skin irritation. We're not doctors, so we can't back up this claim, but what we can say for sure is that probiotics are generally beneficial to the skin.

Super seeds

In developing our babyganics Eczema Lotion, we discovered that on top of the natural and moisturizing ingredients we were already using in our skincare products, when we added a 100 percent natural and balanced blend of cold-pressed seed oils to our solution, our cream wash and lotions became even more soothing and nourishing for a baby's sensitive and developing skin. Turns out the oils from seeds like sunflower, cranberry, red raspberry, tomato, and black cumin are packed with nutrients, vitamins, essential fatty acids, powerful antioxidants, and anti-inflammatory properties that both protect your baby's skin from external damage and nourish it as she grows. All that from a few seeds—who knew? We combined these powerful seed oils and created our exclusive NeoNourish Complex that goes into nearly all of our skincare products, including our disposable diapers.

Q: **Dear Founding Fathers,**

My six-month-old son's pediatrician prescribed hydrocortisone to treat a skin irritation. I totally trust her advice, but I'm not sure I want to use a steroid cream on my son. I've read that steroid creams like hydrocortisone can be very effective at clearing up skin irritations like eczema, but one of the possible side effects includes a weakened immunity, making my baby even more vulnerable to germs and infections in the future. I've also heard steroids can stall my baby's growth and development. I feel like it's a toss-up between a short-term solution and long-term health. What's your advice?

A: **Dear Steroid-Stumped,**

This is a tough call. In a perfect world, we wouldn't have to treat our children's ailments with drugs that could potentially enter their bloodstream and break down their natural defenses to fight infections, but there are medical conditions that legitimately call for the prescribed use of steroids like hydrocortisone. Our fatherly advice: If you can treat the problem without drugs or steroid-based products—fantastic! We believe that in most cases you can smooth out rough patches and even get the best results by adopting a few simple and smart solutions like checking irritants off your laundry list, reducing your child's soak time in the tub, and treating the skin with a drug-free over-the-counter cream or moisturizer that's designed to soothe and calm irritations. If, however, your child's skin irritation persists and your doctor deems a steroid cream necessary, *listen to your doc*! And follow her precise directions! Use the appropriate quantity (no more!) and apply it only for the recommended duration. Steroid cream is not a long-term solution. It is, however, sometimes the only temporary relief.

Perplexed over petroleum

While we're still on the subject of soothing, relieving, and nourishing your baby's dry, itchy skin, we want to say a few more words about petrochemicals. A lot of parents we meet are under the impression that petroleum-filled products like mineral oil and petroleum jelly are great for moisturizing and lubricating skin and soothing cuts, burns, and diaper rash. And while there's nothing inherently unsafe about products with petrochemicals, they're still not necessarily your safest bet. Sure, our parents (and probably yours, too) swore by their big jar of petroleum jelly because it did what it promised to do—it sealed in moisture—and just as important, it was cheap. But when we got into the baby skincare business we learned a few things that our parents hadn't known. While petroleum jelly itself is relatively harmless (in fact, it's been approved by the cosmetic regulatory department of most countries around the world), the chemical process of converting petroleum into usable ingredients that make a product smooth, thick, and jelly-like can create trace amounts of 1,4-Dioxane, a toxic by-product that easily penetrates the skin and is on California's Proposition 65 list of substances known to cause cancer and birth defects. The creation of 1,4-Dioxane doesn't always happen in the manufacturing process of petroleum-filled products, but it can, so when choosing ingredients for our skincare line, we ask ourselves, "Why risk it?" As a parent choosing products for your child's delicate skin, you might ask yourself the same question.

We're big believers in better to be baby-safe than sorry, so if you ask us, the safest way to go is to use products that are petroleum-free, of which there are many great ones. We've found that there are safer alternatives that function just as well (without clogging pores and trapping in dirt and bacteria—a frequent complaint of petroleum jelly and mineral oil) and are more natural, while still soothing to dry, cracked, and irritated skin.

Before we move on, we should also mention baby oil, another favorite for softening and protecting babies' skin. You probably got a bottle or two at your baby shower from a been-there-done-that mother who swears by it. A well-meaning nurse may have even sent some home with you from the hospital. But what you might not know is that the harmless baby oil that your own mother slapped on your behind is basically just mineral oil, *a petroleum-based ingredient.* It coats the skin and not in a good way, but by blocking its ability to breathe, sweat, and release toxins. It's not a great skincare ingredient, especially for thin, super-sensitive and permeable baby skin.

If you like the silky feel of baby oil on your baby's behind, you can easily substitute it with organic coconut, olive, or grape seed oils. These natural vegetable oils work wonders at hydrating sensitive skin and creating a safer protective skin barrier. Natural oils also make an excellent after-bath (or anytime) moisturizer and give a wonderful baby massage! Beeswax, shea butter, and mango butter are masters at soothing irritated skin, including chapped lips and noses.

Be sunsitive

We'd be straight-up bad parents if we didn't mention the importance of sun care. We'll talk more about how to have the most fun in the sun in Step 7, but since we're already on the subject of baby skincare, sunscreen deserves a few minutes in the hot seat.

Q: **Dear Founding Fathers,**

My son is four months old and we're heading into a long hot summer. We have a family vacation planned where we'll spend many days poolside. I feel like I should protect him from the sun, but I read everywhere that infants under six months of age shouldn't wear sunscreen. Help!

A: **Dear Sun Shy,**

You're not the only one confused about sunscreen. Let us shine some light on the truth: The FDA recommends that babies under the age of six months not wear sunscreen, but this is not because sunscreen is any more harmful at that age—it's that the bright sun is extra dangerous to sensitive infant skin. Your baby's delicate face burns faster than an older child's and takes longer to recover. So what the FDA is really saying is: Babies under six months old should not be exposed to the damaging rays of the sun. It's about sun exposure, not sunscreen.

And while we agree with their recommendation, let's be realistic. You're going to occasionally leave the house, go on a picnic, take a vacation (at least, we hope so!). In these situations, the safest solution is to protect your baby with a few precautionary steps—put a hat on his delicate head, dress him in clothes with sun filters, and stick to the shade. If protective clothing and shade aren't available, apply a mineral-based sunscreen to small, exposed areas such as the face and the back of the hands. We recommend a broad-spectrum protection UVA/UVB sunscreen with an SPF of at least 30 that you reapply every two hours, and more frequently if your baby's in the water.

Bathtub Basics

OK . . . who's ready for bath time? A question before we begin: What are you using in the tub? Not what are you using to clean your tub, but what are you using to *clean your baby*? Before your baby's next rub-a-dub-dub, consider what you're using to create all those sudsy-suds. Many popular bath products on the shelves today contain harsh chemicals like phthalates, synthetic fragrances, alcohol, and dyes that can be absorbed into your baby's skin. Some "tear-free" shampoos even contain formaldehyde, a known cancer-causing chemical. Talk about something a concerned parent can really cry about!

Kevin and Keith's
NOT-SO-SAFE-SUDS List

1,4-DIOXANE

Where you'll find it: In foaming and sudsy products like shampoo and bubble bath and petroleum-based products. You will not see 1,4-Dioxane listed in an ingredient list, so your clue is to avoid petroleum-based products or ingredients with "oleth" and "eth" endings like sodium laureth sulfate.

Why it's bad news: 1,4-Dioxane is considered a probable human carcinogen by the EPA. The California EPA also lists 1,4-Dioxane as a suspected kidney toxicant, neurotoxicant, and respiratory toxicant.

DIETHANOLAMINE (DEA), TRIETHANOAMINE (TEA), AND MONOETHANOLAMINE (MEA)

Where you'll find them: In shampoos, soaps, body lotions, shaving creams, and bubble baths.

Why they're bad news: These foaming agents can form cancer-causing nitrates when combined with certain preservatives. They're restricted in Europe, yet are still used in the United States. Americans may be exposed ten to twenty times per day to DEA, TEA, and MEA through personal-care products, and the FDA warns that the risk of exposure is significantly increased for children.

Just as when you shopped for safe bath and tile cleaners, before you put another bottle of foamy, bubbly bath suds in your cart, look for warning labels and check out the ingredient list. The laws for full disclosure are stricter for personal care products than household products and fragrance formulas. All ingredients must be listed and visible to the consumer on the package. But if poring over an ingredient list isn't something you have the time or energy for (hey, we get it; we're busy parents, too!), simply notice what your bottle of bubbles *doesn't* include. Look for shampoos, body washes, and bubble bath with labels that specifically claim to be free of parabens, sulfates, phthalates, petroleum, and toxins like DEA and SLES.

According to Kevin . . .

I remember when we shared one of our first bath products with parents. We used to joke around that the tagline should be, "It's so safe you can drink it," because the truth is, our products *are* safe enough to drink (although we don't recommend it. Bubble bath burps are no fun, trust me!). At one of our first trade shows, our most daring salesperson decided to put it to the test. As people wandered up to our booth, he'd take a BIG swig! At one point, he downed half a bottle. Naturally, this got us a lot of attention, and before we knew it, drinking our babyganics Foaming Shampoo and Bodywash became our thing. Once during an on-camera interview, the photographer took multiple shots of me squirting our bath soap into my mouth. We've shared swigs with several news anchors and many important store buyers. Hey, when you've got a good shtick, you might as well stick to it. And it turns out Hollywood thinks so, too. The movie *The Guilt Trip* is loosely based on the founding of babyganics. The main character, played by Seth Rogen, travels throughout the country drinking his green cleaning product as part of his sales pitch. I taught him everything he knows!

Q: **Dear Founding Fathers,**

My ten-month-old loves bath time. He splashes, wriggles around, and laughs at us, but his absolute favorite thing to do in the bath is to *drink* the bathwater. Should I be worried about him swallowing substances like chlorine in the water?

A: **Dear DWB (Drinking While Bathing),**

The chlorine levels would have to be pretty darn high to be harmful, and if you've installed a home filtering system or even just an individual filter in your bathtub, you shouldn't have to worry about your child swallowing chlorine. The only real concern when it comes to drinking bathwater is whether or not you're using bath products with potentially harmful ingredients that can be ingested.

Assuming your water is clean and your products are safe, sipping suds isn't a huge health concern. In fact, tub time can be a no-fail opportunity to teach your baby a few drinking skills. Fill up a regular plastic cup from the faucet and let him have at it. If he slugs and spills, what's the harm? He's already wet! And while he's working so hard to perfect his new skill, it helps you out, too, because your baby's totally preoccupied while you scrub those hard to reach areas (like underneath that chubby chin!).

Hiney Helpers

Let's turn things around, shall we? We'll now move on to your baby's backside and discuss our approach to diapers, wipes, and everything, hiney-helpful. As with everything you purchase and use, you have choices. In the diaper department, you have lots to consider. We're here to help you do just that.

Consider cloth

OK, we know that asking modern humans—used to modern conveniences—to consider cloth diapers is a tough sell, so we'll just share what we've learned about this option and you decide what makes sense for you and your family.

A Few Great Benefits of
USING CLOTH DIAPERS

- Savings! It's been estimated that your family could save in the $2,500+ range per child, per year. Holy cr*p!
- Less waste. It is also estimated that ten thousand tons of disposable diapers are added to landfills every day. Cloth diapers means less waste you have to haul to the curb.
- Early training. Potty training may be easier and faster. Children raised in cloth diapers typically know what "wet" feels like and choose not to feel that way sooner than their disposable-diapered young friends.
- Always on hand. No more frantic overnight orders from Diapers.com; just throw a load into the washing machine and your baby will be good to go!

If you decide to go with cloth, we recommend cloths made from natural fibers like organic cotton or hemp, which have not been treated with pesticides and chemicals while growing. Terry cloth and thin flannel are also safe materials and feel good on the backside. We're fans of the following brands: bumGenius, Under the Nile, and Fuzbaby.

Flushable inserts

If you like the idea of cloth diapers because they leave a light carbon footprint, but you can't fully commit to all they entail (cloth diapers can be a handful!), consider disposable inserts. These slip into a reusable cloth diaper, and once the insert's been, well, "activated" as they say in the biz, you remove it and flush it down. We like environmentally conscious brands, such as gDiapers and Charlie Banana, that use a biodegradable and plastic-free disposable lining. They're some of the only diapers you can easily flush, compost, or toss.

And while we believe that both cloth diapers and diapers with disposable inserts are great choices from the perspective of protecting your baby's behind *and* the planet she sits on, we're also realists. As young fathers, we understand that convenience is king.

According to Kevin . . .

I was on a family trip to South Carolina, the flight was going really well, and Ali and I thought we might actually pull off a chill trip with two children under the age of four. Not so fast. I suddenly noticed my six-month-old needed a diaper change—big-time. Ryan and I headed to the bathroom, and that's when things got interesting. First, I couldn't figure out where the changing table was, and second, my son was wearing a cloth diaper. What was I supposed to do with the dirty diaper? Take it back to my seat? Hand it to the flight attendant? I won't provide the details of how this story ended. Let's just say I learned the hard way about the occasional benefits of disposable diapers.

The disposable dilemma

As far as we're concerned, parents shouldn't have to choose between the planet or their baby. For years, new parents have debated the convenience of disposable diapers versus their environmental impact, but why not have it both ways? We firmly believe that in the diaper department, you can make purchasing choices that balance practicality with safety and responsibility. In other words—you can choose convenience and still do the right thing. Take it from us, you'll find plenty of things to feel guilty about as a parent as the years go by. We think using a disposable diaper doesn't have to be one of them.

As guys who've gotten into the disposable-diaper-producing business, we're fully aware of their cons—namely, they can be wasteful. A baby goes through an average of 5,000 to 8,000 diaper changes before they move on to undies, and according to the EPA, some disposable diapers take up to 450 years to fully decompose. They can also be expensive to the consumer (you), and many are not so healthy for your baby. Often made with artificial dyes, synthetic fragrances to mask odors, and petrochemicals and plastics in the inner and outer liners, many disposable diapers can irritate one of the most sensitive areas of your baby's skin.

Sure, that's a lot of cons . . . but the good news (actually it's GREAT news) is you don't need all of those unnatural additives to have a disposable diaper that performs really well and is also easy on the environment. Believe it or not, disposable diapers actually have a lot going for them. Check out this list of pros.

A Few GREAT Benefits of Using Disposable Diapers

- Convenience. Disposable diapers are available almost everywhere—your nearest supermarket, big-box store, corner market, baby retailer, and convenience store.
- Longevity. Most disposable diapers hold more than three times the amount of wetness than cloth diapers. This means a whole lot less leaks and diaper changes—and we don't know a mom or dad who doesn't love that!
- Not necessarily *more* wasteful. Disposable diapers have nearly the same environmental impact as reusable cloth diapers when you consider the amount of water and electricity or gas used to wash and dry the cloth diapers regularly.
- Velcro tabs. Disposables are a relative cinch to secure, even with a few wiggles and waggles.
- Day-care friendly. Many day-care centers prefer (some insist on!) disposable diapers.

As parents who understand very well the value of convenience, and as business guys who make baby-safe products, we asked ourselves—Why not create a disposable diaper that's parent-friendly, baby-friendly, eco-friendly, *and* wallet friendly, too? Why shouldn't parents (and our babies) have it all? No good reason! So we created babyganics ultra-absorbent, disposable diapers. They're made from natural and renewable resources and are free of toxins, latex, petroleum-based lotions, and fragrance. They're the diaper of our babies' dreams. (Ours, too!) They arrived in stores just in time for the birth of Ashton Kai Garber, Keith and Nicole's newest addition to the family.

Hey, it's no secret that we're big fans of our babyganics diaper line, but we really do encourage you to shop around until you find the right fit for your baby's behind. The way your baby goes through diapers, you deserve one that's just about perfect. Before choosing a disposable diaper for your baby's behind, consider the smart solutions below.

SMART SOLUTIONS:

Choosing a Safer Disposable Diaper

- Avoid synthetic fragrances and artificial dyes. Some disposable diapers contain synthetic fragrances to mask stinky odors and are colored with dyes to make them more attractive, but neither is beneficial to your baby's sensitive bottom.

- Avoid latex. It can easily cause skin irritation and allergic reactions.
- Choose chemical-free and unbleached. Many disposable diapers are bleached to make them look white, and this bleaching process can create toxic by-products like dioxins, which are dangerous to both our babies and the planet. (Some disposables are dyed a natural beige to look, well, natural, but aren't necessarily any safer than the white ones.)
- Choose biodegradable materials. No disposable diaper is 100 percent biodegradable but when you choose a disposable made with biodegradable materials, you're minimizing your environmental footprint and impact.

Q: **Dear Founding Fathers,**

How do you feel about overnight diapers? I've heard that leaving a superabsorbent diaper on for too long will cause diaper rash and irritate my daughter's skin.

A: **Dear Soppy Sleepovers,**

As a general rule, we don't have a problem with overnight diapers. In fact, if putting an overnight diaper on your infant cuts down on nighttime leaks and helps her (and more importantly—you!) sleep through the night then we're all for it. That decision makes sense.

Naturally, if you leave a superabsorbent diaper on too long it's bound to become irritating (not to mention *heavy*), so as soon as your daughter wakes up in the morning, change her. You might also consider the obvious: If she keeps waking up in the night with a soggy bottom, you may have to move up a diaper size.

It is true that you reduce the probability of diaper rash with more frequent changes, so make a habit of changing your baby's diaper as often as necessary during daytime hours. We say "as necessary" because we've met parents who say they change diapers at the top of every hour to avoid the slightest leak. We've met others who use superabsorbent diapers on long car rides to prolong a rest-stop change. We get the thinking here, but we're not big advocates of either strategy. Overly persistent diaper changes are wasteful, and leaving a superabsorbent diaper on for super-long stretches isn't practical or all that comfortable for your baby.

Treat a tender tush

Once you make the switch to a more natural diaper (chlorine-, latex-, fragrance-, and dye-free) you can expect to see diaper rash less often. Still, we are talking about a really sensitive area here—rashes happen. To help soothe a tender tush or relieve a burning bum, try the smart solutions below.

SMART SOLUTIONS:
Soothe and Relieve

- Air it out. Strip him of his diaper and let him play in the buff. Fresh air does wonders to soothe a tender behind. Because accidents do happen, we recommend putting a blanket down first.
- Use a natural, non-petroleum, plant-based protective ointment at every diaper change and apply generous amounts as a preventative measure. *Ahhh . . . now doesn't that feel better?*
- Choose wipes that are free of chlorine or synthetic fragrances, or simply use paper towels or soft reusable washcloths and warm water.

According to Kevin . . .

Whenever my son Tyler got a diaper rash, I could never quite find the right ointment or cream to soothe it, so Ali and I would often just strip him down and let him run around the house so he could air out and heal. Our "butt-naked" approach to diaper rash became a pretty normal practice in our house. So normal that Tyler often greeted our friends and neighbors at the door in his birthday suit. Sometimes, he'd stand in the doorway and start dancing in place. (But hey, he didn't have a rash!)

Around that time, the babyganics team was lab-testing a plant-based, non-petroleum ointment, and I brought home a sample. We discovered that it relieved Tyler's rash overnight. I was so impressed with this healing ointment that when I was training for my first NYC Marathon, I used it to take care of my runner's chafing. TMI? Maybe, but if you're a runner you understand the importance of a rash-free race!

Q: **Dear Founding Fathers,**

I've always used a baby powder on my baby's bum to soothe rashy skin, but a few mothers in my daughter's playgroup have gotten on my case for this. They say powder isn't safe. Is this true? Now when I use it I feel like a bad mom. Help!

A: **Dear Powder-Perturbed,**

First of all, you've been doing what you thought was best for your baby so you're *not* a bad mom. We are all learning and growing as parents every day . . . so today, here's what you can learn: Diaper rash is best treated with products that moisturize rather than those with ingredients like powder that can dry out and irritate the skin. For this reason, we recommend tossing the baby powder out with the baby oil.

What's safest for your baby? Well, lightweight baby powder floats into the air becoming a dust that your baby may breathe, and some (especially those containing talc) can irritate a baby's lung tissue when inhaled. All said, if you like the powdering ritual, try baking soda or cornstarch (note: cornstarch, not *cornmeal,* you're not making polenta!), which helps soothe diaper rash without drying out the skin like some conventional baby powders. See? You learn something new every day. And *that* is why you're a good mom!

Wipe it good

Just as important as choosing the right diaper for your baby's behind is choosing the healthiest and safest wipes. With frequent diaper changes, you're going through even more wipes (most parents average between two and four for every diaper change), and with every use you're applying whatever ingredients they contain to your child's bare, sensitive skin. Look on any parenting message board and you'll find a post from some disgruntled parent who swears that their wipes made their baby's tushy rash even worse. And they probably have. The reason? Lots of wipes contain the same nasty, irritating ingredients that we've already advised you to stay away from (you can probably say them in unison now): phthalates, parabens, sulfates, chlorine, and bleach. So look for fragrance-free, chlorine-free baby wipes made with natural oils and wipe your wee ones with no worries.

Another consideration: Where do you *store* your wipes? We're big fans of the luxuriously modern baby-wipe warmer (OXO Tot makes a great one with an easy-press dispensing mechanism—super cool!) because it does exactly what it claims to—warms cold and clammy wipes. All of our babies responded well to warm wipes (no surprise there: They're warm!). The thing about a wipe warmer is that it has to be cleaned about once a week with an effective, nontoxic cleaner. Also—and this is key—if your warmer has a sponge at the bottom that stays wet in order to keep the wipes moist, that also needs to be kept clean. Warm, moist sponge + dark, enclosed location = bacteria! Our fatherly advice: If you're down to the last wipe and can see the sponge at the bottom of the warmer, it's time to take it out and wash it good. In addition to regular cleanings, replace the sponge every few months.

OK, clean baby? Check! Skin is nourished and protected? Check! But all work and no play makes for . . . well, for one thing it makes for bored parents. So, let's talk playtime! Next up, we'll advise you on how to encourage your baby to have fun, play, and thrive safely inside the home.

Step 3: Baby Body

Smart Solutions at a Glance

Fine and Handy

- Teach good hand washing at an early age with simple soap and water.
- Prevent sickness by teaching your child to avoid touching his eyes, nose, and mouth.
- Minimize the spread of germs by teaching your child to cover her sneezes and coughs.
- Use alcohol-free, nontoxic hand wipes when soap and water isn't available.

Kissy Face

- Hydrating and moisturizing from day one is an absolute must. Avoid products with artificial dye, synthetic fragrances, and alcohol.
- Use a UVA/UVB sunscreen with an SPF of at least 30 that you reapply every two hours, and more frequently if your baby's in the water.
- If you haven't yet made the switch to a natural, fragrance-free laundry detergent, now's the time!

Bathtub Basics

- After bath, apply a generous amount of non-petroleum-based cream or emollient to red and inflamed dry areas to seal in moisture and soothe eczema.
- Consider cutting tub time back to two or three times a week, keep your baby's bathwater cool, and reduce the overall soak time.
- Look for shampoos, body washes, and bubble bath with labels that specifically claim to be free of DEA, TEA, MEA, sulfates, and harsh chemicals or toxins.

Hiney Helpers

- When choosing a cloth diaper, choose natural fibers like organic cotton or hemp, or terry cloth and thin flannel, that are safe and feel good on the skin.

- When choosing a disposable diaper, avoid latex, synthetic fragrances, and artificial dyes. Choose diapers that are unbleached and made with biodegradable materials.
- To relieve a tender tushy, use a natural, non-petroleum, plant-based protective ointment at every diaper change and apply generous amounts as a preventative measure.
- Choose wipes that are bleach-, chlorine-, paraben-, sulfate-, and phthalate-free.

Step 4

Safe Play

It's time we had a playdate! Being just a bit more informed than you already are about the toys, gadgets, and gear on the market today means you can start to make decisions that will keep your child safe without making play any less fun. In this step, we'll share with you what we've learned about

- Warning labels
- Playing safe in toyland

- The nuts and bolts of baby gear
- Taking a balanced approach to screen time

Warning labels

Playtime should be fun, not an occasion for parents to worry, but the worrisome truth is that just because a toy's on the market doesn't mean that it's been tested or that it meets government safety standards. The U.S. Consumer Product Safety Commission (CPSC) does its best to test for safety and enforce federal standards, but it's just a fact that some toys slip through the cracks and into your child's toy box. This is why you frequently hear about toy recalls.

So what's a cautious parent supposed to do? You can start by learning to identify the kinds of toys that should be off-limits so you can choose safer alternatives. Again, simple awareness goes a long way. When it comes to toys and gear that may be classified as dangerous or hazardous because of the materials used to make them, we're here to help you ID the toxic offenders. Check out the list below for an example of what we're most concerned about.

Kevin and Keith's NOT-SO-FUN List

POLYVINYL CHLORIDE (PVC)

Where you'll find it: Plastic toys, food packaging, shower curtains, and building materials. PVC is often found in baby gear like car seats, high chairs, and infant strollers.

Why it's bad news: Vinyl chloride, the chemical used to make PVC plastic, is a known human carcinogen that's also been linked to hormone disruption and birth defects. You can be exposed to PVC by eating food or drinking water contaminated with it. Yes, sucking on a toy made with PVC plastic totally counts! You and your baby can also be exposed by inhaling it. Smell that strong, fresh-from-the-package scent? One PVC shower curtain, for example, can release as many as 108 volatile organic chemicals into the air. Some of these VOCs can cause developmental damage as well as upset the central nervous, respiratory, and reproductive systems.

PHTHALATES

Where you'll find them: Phthalates are chemicals commonly used in PVC plastic to make toys extra squishy, inflatable, and flexible. Phthalates are the stuff that makes toys so irresistible to babies who love to suck and chew.

Since 2009, the United States and Canada have required that toys like teethers and pacifiers that go into a child's mouth be phthalate-free. Note: This rule doesn't cover *all* toys, even though sooner or later most toys end up in the mouth.

Why they're bad news: Phthalates can leach out of PVC plastic when your baby mouths them, and are linked to hormone disruption, reproductive and developmental problems, and cancer.

BISPHENOL A (BPA)

Where you'll find it: BPA is a plasticizer used to make plastic toys soft and flexible.

Why it's bad news: BPA can leach out of plastic when heated, so when toys go into the mouth (and again, what toy doesn't?), your child is at risk of exposure. BPA has been associated with poor sperm count, early puberty, breast cancer, obesity, diabetes, and ADHD.

LEAD

Where you'll find it: Lead can be prevalent in painted toys, especially those imported from China, India, and Mexico. In 1978, lead was banned in house paint, on products marketed specifically to children, and in dishes and cookware in the United States; however, it is still widely used in other countries. It may also be found in older toys made in the United States before the ban. Note: The use of lead in plastics has not been banned. Lead is often used as a stabilizer in PVC plastic. Its use is somewhat regulated in products made in the United States, but again, not in imported PVC products. One study found lead levels 30 to 100 times higher in imported toys than the federal limit for lead in children's items.

Why it's bad news: If inhaled or ingested by licking, gumming, or chewing, lead can damage the developing brain and nervous system of your child. Lead exposure has been linked to memory loss, learning problems, and ADHD.

Agreed, this info doesn't sound like fun, but not to worry. Most of these nasty chemicals are pretty easy to avoid once you know how and where to look for them. Take lead, for example. Understanding that lead is almost nonexistent in newer toys made in this country, skip the antiques stores, garage and estate sales, and politely decline hand-me-down toys from the last generation.

According to Kevin . . .

When I learned about the potential health risks of BPA, PVC, and phthalates in plastic toys, I was not a happy guy. I hated that I might be exposing my own kids to dangerous chemicals, but also the thought of removing all the plastic toys from my kids' toy bin made my head hurt.

Ali and I decided to take a less extreme and somewhat relaxed approach. Instead of focusing on what they couldn't play with, we were just pickier about what we *did* allow them to play with. We slowly weeded out the toys we didn't feel good about and the boys hardly missed them. Sure, this gets harder to do as your kids get older and you have less control, but when they're infants and toddlers, it's pretty easy to make their toy choices for them. Ali and I also believe that by just keeping the number of toys in the house to a minimum, our kids appreciate even more all the cool stuff they already have. As an added bonus, there's less for us to trip over and clean up!

Yeah, in a perfect world, Ali and I would prefer that Tyler and Ryan never come into contact with toys that contain PVC and BPA, but the reality is that it's nearly impossible to avoid plastic altogether. And there are actually a lot of very cool toys out there made with safe plastics. So rather than becoming toy extremists, we just do our best to introduce toys into their world that do the least harm, are healthy and safe and . . . *give them the freedom to have fun*!

SMART SOLUTIONS:
Choosing the Safest Toys

- Buy PVC-free. Seek out toys clearly labeled this way. If a toy is not clearly marked "PVC-free," look on the packaging for a 1, 2, 4, or 5 next to the three-arrow recycling symbol. These codes indicate PVC-free. If it's marked 3, put it back on the shelf. Number 3 means PVC!

- Buy BPA-free. Seek out toys clearly labeled "BPA-free." Again, if it's not clearly marked, look for toys with a recycle code of 1, 2, 4, or 5. If it's marked 7 put it back on the shelf. Number 7 means BPA!
- Buy new-ish. The United States and Canada require that toys that can be put into the mouth (teething toys and pacifiers, specifically) be phthalate-free, and legislation that took effect in 2009 puts even heavier restrictions on phthalates and lead use in toys.
- Buy "Made in the USA." Not only is this good for the economy, but homegrown toys made after 2007 are likely lead-free. If you're buying toys that have been painted, look for "nontoxic" and "lead-free" labels.
- Buy established and reputable brands. Brand-name toy makers and retailers don't want to suffer a toy recall—it's bad for business. The stakes aren't as high for off-brand and imported toys sold in discount stores.
- Buy low-odor and nontoxic. Choose water-based markers, pens, and paints for your little artist that are labeled "low-odor" or "nontoxic" or that are approved by the Art & Creative Materials Institute. The ACMI-approved product seal "AP," indicates that the product has been evaluated by a qualified toxicologist and is labeled in accordance with federal and state laws. For obvious reasons, avoid art supplies that say "harmful or fatal if swallowed." If the product isn't clearly marked and you're not sure how safe it is, do the smell test. Do the markers stink? Does the paint give you a head-rush? If the answer is yes, postpone arts and crafts day until you have safer supplies to work with.
- Buy natural fibers. Instant comfort and security that's also safe is a

stuffed animal made with natural, organic fibers and colored with nontoxic dyes.

- Buy wood. Natural, unfinished, and solid-wood toys or those decorated with nontoxic paints and natural finishes are a great way to go.

In addition to implementing the smart solutions above, consider using this recommended checklist of questions we often ask ourselves when shopping for the safest toys on the block. (As for specific brands and toys we like, there's a long list in the coming pages.)

Is the toy on my kid's level?

Most toy packaging includes a "recommended age" sticker to give you a solid starting point for judging whether it's appropriate for your kid. A toy labeled "3+," for example, is not going to be the safest choice for your newborn. Consider, too, that every child learns differently and only you know what level your kid's truly operating on. Be realistic about what he can and cannot do. If that Nerf basketball hoop is over your child's head—both figuratively and literally—put it on the shelf until she grows into it. No harm done!

Does the toy pass the TP test?

Choking on small balls, coins, marbles, and deflated balloons continues to be the most frequent causes of toy-related deaths and ER visits, so until your child turns well past three, toy parts should be bigger than his mouth. Because some mouths are bigger than others (ain't that the truth!), determine whether a toy is safe by putting it through the toilet-paper-roll test: If it can easily slip inside and through a toilet paper roll, it's too small. Toss it out with the rest of the trash—or, again, shelve it for a few years.

Is the toy too heavy?

Could your baby be hurt if the toy fell on her? If so, give it a heave-ho. And if it's broken, fix it! Toys should be well made, securely put together, and free of buttons, yarn, ribbons, beads, zippers—basically anything your child could easily yank, snap, chew off, and swallow. It also goes without saying that toys with sharp edges and points aren't the safest choices for fragile babies and clumsy toddlers.

Does the toy have strings attached?

Be really careful about toys with strings that your child could wrap around her neck. Strings longer than twelve inches are too long!

Is the toy magnetic?

Toys with magnets are often recalled due to their potential safety risks. In fact, the CPSC recommends keeping toys with magnets, especially small ones that can be swallowed, away from children under six years old.

Does the toy run on batteries?

Battery-operated isn't inherently bad. The problem is when batteries or battery fluid ends up in your child's mouth, which could lead to choking, chemical burns, and internal bleeding. Be sure the battery case on that remote control car is secure (screws, duct tape—do what you have to do!) so little hands can't easily pry it open.

How noisy *is* it?

Not only can buzzing, beeping, talking toys drive sane (and tired!) parents crazy, but they can cause hearing loss. Say what? Yup, it's been discovered that one in five children in the United States will have some degree of hearing loss by the time they reach age twelve, and early hearing loss can significantly slow down speech development. If a toy is labeled for "outdoor use," it means it's *too loud*! The next time it starts honking in the middle of the night, you have our permission to turn it off—for good.

Babes in (Safe) Toyland

At this point, you may be thinking, "Note to self: never invite these guys to a party. They take all the fun out of playtime." Not true! We're all about creating an environment that gives babies the freedom to safely learn, explore, and also have tons of fun. So . . . let's start having some! Here's a sampling of toys that are healthy, safe, *and* FUN.

Musical toys (not the same as *noisy* toys): After listening only to Mom's strong and steady heartbeat for nine months, babies enter this world as naturally musical creatures! Not only do musical toys like drums, bells, and mini tambourines make babies feel happy and secure, but as an added bonus, they help with brain development. Some research suggests that music may be more engaging to our babies than speech.

Blocks: We're a little old school but trust us, building blocks never go out of style. Count 'em, stack 'em, knock 'em down—blocks teach eye–hand coordination, inspire creativity, and are a safe, easy way to have a good time. Look for uncolored, unvarnished wood blocks, or colored blocks with nontoxic paints and dyes that don't easily chip.

A plush pal: Whether your child is going to a new caregiver for the first time, a doctor's appointment, or transitioning to a new sleeping arrangement, a plush pal can provide comfort and security. Look for toys made from natural fibers and nontoxic dyes and without buttons that can easily be nibbled off because your child will likely chew on her new pal. Remove plush toys before bedtime—babies should not sleep with *anything* in their cribs. Give all toys a home outside the crib until your pediatrician declares them safe for sleepovers.

A soft ball: Balls help to improve eye–hand coordination and encourage our little ones to become social creatures. A game of toss is a great way to make a new friend at the playground. Shop for balls that are made out of rubber and are free of PVC and BPA.

Books: Most all babies and young children love books. In fact, story time is something your child can begin enjoying in the womb! Did you know that babies tend to prefer books you read aloud to them when you were pregnant? And once they can get their hands on them, chew on the pages or make up their own stories to go with the pictures, books can provide hours of entertainment. Plus, they're one of the safest and healthiest ways for your child to pass her time. When you read to your child every day, you share quality bonding time and help them develop their vocabulary and early literacy skills.

According to Kevin . . .

When Tyler was a baby he had a stuffed elephant that he couldn't sleep without. He sucked on that elephant until he fell asleep at every nap and bedtime. The first time the family went on vacation, Ali and I made a rookie mistake: We forgot his elephant. You've never seen two parents more panicked! The whole car ride, we kept looking at each other: "Why didn't you bring it?" "Why didn't YOU bring it?" We were convinced that without that elephant, Tyler would just stay awake for the rest of his life. When we got to the hotel and set up his crib and settled him in for the night we were beyond stressed. You can guess what happened next. He fell asleep with no problem at all. We couldn't help but laugh at our crazy neurotic behavior. Clearly, we were the ones hooked on that elephant. This story taught us to really ask ourselves when we get stressed, Is this about the kids? Or is this really *our* elephant?

Q: Dear Founding Fathers,

How do you feel about "gently used" toys? I find I can score some pretty good deals at garage sales, thrift stores, and secondhand stores. But I always wonder if they're safe. Thoughts?

A: Dear Used-Confused,

Secondhand toys are a great way to keep costs down. Just be sure to consider safety along with the low price. Approach secondhand toys the same way you would new toys—check that whatever you're about to put into your child's hands is free of pieces that can be easily yanked, snapped, or chewed off. This is especially important with toys that you buy secondhand or have been "regifted" to you by friends and relatives who, c'mon, probably just wanted to unload some stuff! This isn't normally an issue when buying from a baby consignment store; their quality standards are pretty high.

In addition to how it looks on the outside, consider what it's made of on the inside. A toy may look like it's in great shape, but if it was made

Toys We Love and Trust

Most of these toys can be purchased directly from the manufacturer and also from big online retailers like Amazon.com, Diapers.com, Target.com, and Toysrus.com.

Apple Park (www.applepark.com)

Plush toys and teethers for infants and toddlers that are safe for your baby and for the environment. They even have backpacks for school-age kids that are made from 100 percent recycled materials.

B. Toys (justb-byou.com)

B. Toys uses recycled materials (code 1) in its products and packaging, soy-based inks, and water-based varnishes.

Blabla (www.blablakids.com)

Blabla makes lil' things like rattles, puppets, dolls, mobiles, and beanbag chairs made from 100 percent cotton and nontoxic materials.

Child Trek (www.childtrek.com)
Early learning, push and pull, musical, and kitchen toys that use sustainable woods, nontoxic and water-based paints, and formaldehyde-free glue.

Crocodile Creek (www.crocodilecreek.com)
Crocodile Creek specializes in a wide range of toys made of 100 percent rubber and contain no lead, PVC, or BPA.

Green Toys (www.greentoys.com)
Green Toys offers a variety of eco-friendly and nontoxic toys, all of which are free of BPA, phthalates, lead, and other potentially harmful materials. The toys are made in California using recycled milk jugs and are for both outdoor playtime (jump ropes and dump trucks) and indoor use (tea sets, dining sets, and cookware).

before 2009 it's not worth the risk. It may contain phthalates, lead, and other chemicals that have since been banned.

Toys that clean up

Before we move on from baby-safe toys to advising you on the best baby gear, we want to share with you our favorite tips for keeping toys clean. Hey, we're into clean, and your baby is going to spend a lot of time touching and sleeping with (even teething on!) her toys. And that's a good thing! So make sure they're clean enough to . . . uh, chew?

As we mentioned before, nasty cold and flu germs can live on surfaces for minutes or hours and this goes for toys, too. And because most babies play with their food and put toys in their mouths, it's a safe idea to clean them on a regular basis—especially if you're someone who regularly has other kids over at your house grabbing for, playing with, and sucking on the same toys. Germ fest!

According to Kevin . . .

If you're like us, you might not be giving a lot of thought to cleaning the floating alphabet letters and inflatable books in your baby's bath. C'mon, they're in the bath getting soaped up and rinsed off every night along with baby. They're clean, right? Well, it depends on what you do with those bath toys once bath time is over. I'll tell you what Ali and I used to do—we'd either leave them at the bottom of the tub or if we were feeling super organized, we'd jam all of them into a bucket or a net bag to hang overnight. The problem? These soggy toys weren't drying before the boys' next bath, and they were going right back into Tyler's and Ryan's hands and mouths. One day we noticed that the crevices in each of these toys were filled with mold and mildew. No wonder. They were hanging out in the same gunk and grime that collects at the bottom of the tub.

We quickly changed our bath-time routine. Now, when the boys get out of the tub, one of us stays behind and throws all the toys into the bathroom sink, fills it up with soap and water,

Indestructibles (www.indestructiblesinc.com)
Indestructibles makes books built for the way babies read (i.e., with their mouths). They are waterproof, tear-resistant, and baby-durable and are free of BPA, phthalates, PVC, and lead.

Melissa and Doug (www.melissaanddoug.com)
Melissa and Doug manufactures a wide range of baby, toddler, and children's toys, from soft baby toys to puzzles, dollhouses, and trains and other vehicles. The company is dedicated to creating safe toys for all ages and has a product safety sheet for each toy.

Greenpoint Brands (www.mlyim.com)
Greenpont offers a large collection of adorable plush toys and knit toys and a wide range of infant accessories, including stacker toys, stroller toys, plush rattles, knit teethers, and blankets, all made of 100 percent organic cotton.

P'kolino (www.pkolino.com)
P'kolino makes wooden stacking toys, wooden puzzles, and multifunctional art easels made with a plywood base and nontoxic paint finishes.

PlanToys (www.plantoys.com)
PlanToys makes eco-friendly, nontoxic wooden toys using only earth-friendly materials such as chemical-free rubberwood, nontoxic glue, water-based paints and dyes, and recycled materials in its green manufacturing processes (they use solar power primarily). The company makes toys for babies and preschool-age kids (check out their toddler-size "washing machine").

Under the Nile (www.underthenile.com)
Under the Nile sells soft baby toys made of organic cotton.

Vulli (www.Vulli-toys.com)
Vulli makes a wide range of natural rubber teething toys, all of which are free of PVC, phthalates, and BPA.

gives the toys a good scrubbing, rinses them thoroughly, and sets them out to dry. Yeah, this extends bath time (at least for one parent), but the upside is that your kids aren't shoving a pile of gross toys into their mouths. And speaking of a pile of toys, once we started this new routine we realized how many bath toys they had—over thirty! Kind of ridiculous, right? So, we cut it back to three apiece. Not only does this make for a faster cleanup, but it's fewer slimy toys to whack Daddy in the face with.

SMART SOLUTIONS:
Keeping Toys Clean

- Wash and rinse thoroughly. Get in the habit of giving the toys that are most frequently in play a good wash in the sink. A natural dish soap (no parabens, sulfates, or phthalates) with water will do, or wipe them down with an alcohol-free sanitizer. No grime, toxic chemicals, or synthetic fragrances left behind. Let the games begin!
- Run a load. The dishwasher isn't just for casserole dishes. Throw those rubber ducks into the mix.
- Dry them out. A wet, soggy toy is an open invitation for mold and bacteria, so keep toys dry and the mildew away! After washing and rinsing them, set them out to dry on a nearby counter or bath towel.
- High heat. Once a week, throw your child's favorite loveys and stuffed animals in the dryer on high. This will stop any dust mites (more on

Helpful Resource:
Toy Recall

Before buying a new or used toy, consider this: Not all retailers pull recalled toys off shelves in a timely manner, so while it's a bit of a hassle, we suggest doing a quick online search to be sure that the toy you're about to purchase is safe. The following sites feature the latest recall info and are great resources for child safety in general.

www.babycenter.com
www.babyzone.com
www.cpsc.gov
www.parents.com
safemama.com

these allergy- and asthma-provoking critters in Step 6) that have burrowed into their fur from getting too comfortable.

- Less clutter, less grime. The simple truth is that when you limit the number of toys on the floor, you have fewer to trip over and clean.
- Buy washable. Make cleanup easy and buy washable toys.

First Gear

You know where we're going next: All that stuff you tote around requires regular cleaning, too. Between the stroller, the car seat, the sling, and the saucer (seriously, how can such a little person need so much stuff!), all it takes is a little soap and water or a nontoxic cleaner and your job's pretty much done. You're good to go from high to low!

Helpful Resources: The 411 on Safe Gear

For ratings and general info on the safety and effectiveness of a product, check out any of these sites for potential risks before buying:

www.babygearlab.com
www.consumerreports.org
www.healthystuff.org
www.NHTSA.gov

And while we know a thing or two about how to keep things squeaky clean, we don't claim to be product reviewers. In the arena of baby gear, we're consumers just like you, so we're going to leave it to the experts to give you the best recommendations and a definitive thumbs-up or thumbs-down on specific brands. What we *will* share with you are our tips and tricks when shopping for your baby's first gear.

Be prepared. With all the products out there, it won't take long before your living room resembles a My Gym, but there are only a few things you actually need—a car seat, a high chair, and a stroller. As tempting as it may be to bring home the latest, most stylish products out there (admit it: Even when it comes to baby gear, you're still swayed by fashion), we've learned that, while basing our purchasing decisions on practicality and versatility might be a little square, it's the best way to go. That said, no product is perfect, but as two guys who deal every day with some of the biggest retailers and manufacturers out there, we can vouch for the fact that a tremendous effort is being made to design products that are safer and easier to use. Still, it's smart to look into the safest, most practical products available today. Do some online research. Make sure you're up to date on the latest recalls. Ask trusted friends and family to share their knowledge, and then make purchasing decisions that you feel are the most safe. That's really the best you can do.

The lowdown on high chairs

Since your high chair has to hold up for about two years of heavy-duty abuse, you want to be sure you have a model that's safe, sturdy, and simple to clean. The best high chairs have a wide, solid base with a five-point safety strap to keep your baby in place. We all wonder at the beginning if babies really need to be strapped in that securely. *My baby's just eating mashed avocado, not flying to the moon!* But you'll learn pretty quickly that, well, babies move fast and are disarmingly strong. And every baby, at some point, decides that wriggling out of the chair is a game. Why risk it? A five-point safety strap will give you peace of mind that your baby isn't going anywhere.

We also recommend chairs made from durable, high-quality natural wood using nontoxic glue, lead-free finishes, and low-VOC paint. And since you'll find your baby facedown, licking the tray more often than you can imagine, shop for plastic tray covers that are BPA- and phthalate-free and seat cushions that are PBDE-free.

You might also investigate "transition chairs" that safely grow with your child. Some of these height-adjustable chairs can hold up to seventy-nine pounds—the size of a fourth grader! Finally, we recommend shopping for a high chair that's easy to clean. You won't believe how bad yesterday's delicious bean burrito smells when it is left lodged in those hard-to-reach cracks and creases of your baby's seat. Look for chairs with trays and seat covers that can be removed and washed easily.

SMART SOLUTIONS:
Basic High Chair Dos and Don'ts

- Use the safety strap—at every meal. Knowing that she will not wiggle loose and fall will help settle your stomach.
- Don't leave your baby unattended. Even when safely strapped in, kids still wiggle around (if there's a will to be free, there's a way!). Also, at the

rate kids shove food into their mouths, it's important you're right there in case those pureed peas go down the wrong pipe.

- The feeding tray doesn't substitute as a strap. Little fingers are great manipulators, so don't be surprised when your baby learns to pop off the tray. When this happens and he's not securely strapped in, he could easily fall.
- Look for the JPMA certification seal. This means that the manufacturer voluntarily submitted their product(s) for testing and met the highest safety standards for materials, products, systems and services. Bottom line: It's safe.
- Hook it. If you're buying a hook-on chair, make sure the hooking device is strong and the table to which you're attaching it is stable and sturdy enough to hold your baby. (We once met parents who weighed their table base down with a thirty-pound steel anvil to prevent their willful baby from tipping the table over!)

Buckle up

Shopping for car seats can be one of the most frustrating baby-gear-purchasing decisions you'll make because there are countless options and just as many opinions about which are the best. Still, you have to have one. It's not just safe, it's the law. All fifty states require that babies up to eighteen months ride in car seats, and most have laws requiring car seats until a child is at least three years old. The seats you purchase (yup, plural as you'll probably need at least two as your baby grows) often carry a hefty price tag but they really are an investment in safety. Studies show that children who don't ride in car seats are up to four times more likely to be seriously injured in a car crash, and not necessarily on the highway but when simply backing out of the Babies"R"Us parking lot.

So, how do you go about choosing the right one? Our fatherly advice is both general and specific: Buy new. All car seats currently on the market meet the U.S. government's crash- and fire-safety standards (and these standards have gotten stricter over time, in response to research), so any car seat you buy new is technically safe. The best models come with head and side panels that you can adjust up and out for customized, side-impact protection. Still, look for car seats that are free of PBDEs, a class of flame retardant chemicals used in the lining and seat cushion, and PVC plastic. The inside of your car is exposed to heat and UV rays, both of which can accelerate the breakdown of plastic and possibly increase its toxicity.

In recent years many baby products such as car seats, mattress pads, and breast-feeding pillows containing PBDEs have been taken off the market. Many companies such as Wal-Mart, Ikea, and Sam's Club have eliminated PBDEs from many of their products and have realized they can make a fire-safe product without using unsafe chemicals. Still, look for gear labeled "PBDE-free" and stuffed with cotton, polyester, or wool instead of foam.

Even if a car seat meets the federal government's standards and is also chemical-free, it can still be a safety problem if it's installed or used incorrectly. Turns out seven out of ten kids aren't properly buckled in. Make sure your child's not one of them. Consider our smart solutions below before taking your baby for a ride.

SMART SOLUTIONS:
Basic Car Seat Credo

- Install it properly. Before attempting to install your car seat only to get frustrated and declare *This *8! doesn't work,* read the installation guidelines in your owner's manual. Take a deep breath and proceed as directed.
- Practice makes perfect. Remove and reinstall it until you can do it with your eyes shut. (Or with a thousand other things on your mind!)
- Don't turn your baby until you have to. The safest position for your child is in the middle of the back seat facing the rear. If your middle seat has a hump or a pull-down divider and you can't tightly install the base, secure it to either the left- or right-side seat. Wherever it ends up, keep your baby facing the rear for *as long as possible*. The AAP (American Academy of Pediatrics) recommends that children sit facing the rear until the age of two or when he or she reaches and exceeds the maximum weight limit (typically thirty-five pounds) and height limit of the seat. You'll know your child's outgrown his seat when his head is within an inch of the top edge and his shoulders are above the top set of the harness-strap slots. The AAP explains that children are safer facing the rear because in a frontal collision, the stress on a forward-facing child's neck can more easily injure the spine. (By age four your child will likely have outgrown his front-facing seat. Check with your state regarding the safety regulations for belt-positioning booster seats.)

- Tighten up. Your goal is to get the tightest possible fit with the least amount of give.
- Lock up. It's always a good idea to keep car doors and windows locked while driving, especially those closest to curious little baby hands.
- Consider a window shade. This isn't necessary, but it's a nice thing to have. You don't like to be blasted by the sun, and neither does your baby!
- Air it out. Park your baby's car seat outside for a few days before installing it so that any toxic chemicals that might be lingering in the materials have a chance to off-gas.

Q: **Dear Founding Fathers,**

My neighbor offered us her used car seat and I'm tempted to accept. It looks to be in excellent condition. Her son rode in it safely until he transitioned to a booster seat and accepting her hand-me-down would save us a few hundred dollars. Can this be an exception to your "buy new" rule?

A: **Dear Question the Exception,**

Your request for an exception has been . . . uh, tentatively granted. When it comes to car seats, if you're not buying new, our advice is to make sure it's in *very* good condition. Be wary of ripped lining, exposed foam, or anything that appears to be breaking down. Make sure it was made in the last five years and hasn't been recalled for safety violations. Older car seats were designed to meet outdated safety standards, especially in regard to the use of toxic chemicals in the plastic, cushion, and lining. So even if it looks good as new, if it's been collecting dust for a few years, we suggest you pass. Another consideration—be sure it comes with the instruction manual so that you can confidently install it. If your neighbor no longer has it, see if you can find it online or call the company. Most manufacturers will happily send you one free of charge. Finally, be sure it has all its original parts, has not been in a crash, and comes from someone you trust. So our answer is a qualified . . . *maybe*?

Helpful Resource: *Install an Expert*

Feeling car-seat challenged? No problem. Call a CPST. A certified child-passenger safety technician can check your car seat installation for you. Appointments take only about thirty minutes and they're free! Go to www.seatcheck.org and type in your zip code to find the nearest inspection locations—there are more than thirty-three thousand CPSTs nationwide.

Stroller sanity

There's the snap-and-go, the jogging stroller, the car stroller, the double stroller, the double jogging stroller, and the umbrella stroller—*help!* Aside from choosing a style, model, and brand that fits your family's needs, how do you also choose the one that's safest for your baby? First of all, relax. Choosing a stroller can be an overwhelming (and, expensive) undertaking. But know that you can count on most stroller manufacturers to make a safe product. It's just a matter of what features you want, how much luxury you desire, and how much you're willing to spend.

As with all things baby, before making your purchase, consider first what it's made from. We favor a stroller manufactured with PVC- and phthalate-free plastic and with fabrics made from organic fibers free of flame-retardant chemicals like PBDEs. We also like removable and washable fabrics, since wherever your baby strolls, grime will likely hitch a ride. When it comes to sunshades, look for one that actually blocks the sun. (You'd be amazed by how many don't!) Find a canopy with UPF protection. Other safety considerations are maneuverability and brake control. Do a few test-drives. You should be able to push your stroller in a straight line one-handed (and do the Hokey Pokey and turn yourself around). Look for strollers with swivel wheels in the front and back that lock when you put on the brakes. Finally, does the seat recline? Newborns need to chill in a nearly flat position for at least six months before they have the neck and head control to sit up and take a look around.

SMART SOLUTIONS:

Basic Stroller Dos and Don'ts

- Use the safety strap—for every stroll. A secure strap is a must and, as with high chairs, we recommend a five-point harness that wraps around the waist, and secures between the legs and down over the shoulders.
- Lock it into place. Avoid getting the side-eye (you *know* the side-eye) when your stroller folds up like an accordion with your child inside. This is especially embarrassing when it happens in line at Starbucks . . . not that we're, uh, speaking from experience.

- JPMA certified. Look for a stroller that's been certified by the Juvenile Products Manufacturers Association to ensure it meets current safety standards.
- Recycle and Reuse. When the time comes to part ways with your stroller (you should get a few good years out of it), consider passing it on rather than storing it in a dark corner of the garage or basement. Some stroller companies actually have recycling and donation programs where they'll repair, refurbish, and clean your used stroller before donating it to a family in need.

OK, that's our short list of baby-gear must-haves. As for all the other stuff, we'll leave that to you. Even though there are only a few things on our list, these purchases can really add up, so before you make the investment, consider registering for these items. A car seat is a perfect baby-shower gift. Grandparents and godparents love to go in on these big-ticket items. But don't leave the research to the gift givers. Be specific. Ask for the brands and models you've decided are the safest and best for your needs.

An e-Motional Debate

Let's spend a few minutes discussing a debate that can get a little heated between those who find the latest educational technology and media a must-have for the modern baby and those who are on the e-fence. What are the potential health and safety risks of TVs, smartphone apps, computer games, and tablets? When can you safely introduce them to your child? If you're like us, you have *no clue*! All we know for sure is that once kids tune in, good luck trying to get them to tune out. We often see babies (yes, we're talking *babies*) playing games and watching shows on their parents' iPads or smartphones, or sometimes their own! They are mesmerized, and their parents, naturally, are grateful for the relief. So on this we defer to the experts at the American Academy of Pediatrics.

According to their most recent research, your child can begin to safely engage in "screen time" starting at age two, and they recommend limiting that time to two hours a day. They make a good argument that while many educational shows and electronic toys can help toddlers learn, screen time is a passive way of learning. A stacking and nesting app on your iPad, for example, doesn't engage your child's senses in quite the same way or require the same amount of creativity and problem solving as stacking *actual blocks*. It turns out that when passive screen time replaces real-world playtime, the brain is less engaged. Active, imaginative playtime, on the other hand, stimulates, challenges, and develops the brain. What's more, educational shows are often lost on children under two. Watching cartoon characters sing the alphabet might be entertaining, but it's not necessarily teaching your child anything. Babies and toddlers under two are simply too young to understand what's happening on screen and are much better off learning directly from you—the flesh and blood parent in the room. The AAP has also found that screen time cuts down on beneficial "talk time" where you and your child discuss the activity at hand. Talk time is invaluable for teaching your child critical problem solving, language, and social skills. It's also important quality time spent together.

While we agree with the AAP's recommendation, we know that tuning out in today's electronic culture is nearly impossible. The reality is that many kids have unlimited access to technology and engage in some form of media every day, and as our kids get older, it may be that the technology they're playing with today will become more and more relevant to their productivity, both personally and professionally. Our fatherly advice: try to strike a healthy balance. Don't go nuts trying to keep electronics away from your kids. But set some safe and healthy limits.

According to Kevin . . .

Our boys are four and seven and are in school for the majority of the day. During their off-time, Ali and I have structured their play time this way: Instead of saying, "You only have two hours of screen time," we encourage them to engage in activities that don't involve screens for just two hours a day. Pretty tricky, huh? In our house, this means staying away from TVs, computers, iPad, iPhone, iPod touch, Nintendo 3DS, and Wii (yeah, we're pretty plugged in) for a two-hour window where they must do *something else.* So far, this reverse psychology has worked (we'll keep you posted). When the weather's good, they play outside with their friends for two hours and stumble in for dinner. Once plates are cleared and homework is done, they can plug in without a word of protest from us. Before you know it—it's bedtime and they haven't spent more than a couple of hours in front of a screen. Sure, it becomes more of a challenge during bad weather and winter months. That's when parents have to step in and create distractions as tempting as their electronics. (Baking? Bowling? Monopoly??) Not always an easy task.

SMART SOLUTIONS:

Creating Healthy Screen Time

- No screen time until the age of two. Until then, your child is simply too young to understand what's happening on screen and is much better off learning directly from you.
- Enforce two hours a day. Limit screen time to two hours a day for children two years old and older.
- Watch and learn together. When you sit and watch shows together, not only can you monitor what your child is watching, but you're also right there to discuss what you're seeing and answer any questions your child might have about content. This makes for quality learning time.
- Protect the eyes. Many pediatric optometrists warn that prolonged screen time (on handheld devices particularly, where children's eyes are focused up close) causes children to strain their eyes in a way that may compromise healthy vision. Try to keep screens an arm's length away from your child and encourage screen time breaks, where he focuses on

something far away for at least twenty to thirty seconds before returning his focus to the screen.

- Skip the commercials. You know the ones we're talking about—commercials that are sexually suggestive, violent, aggressive, or confusing to a young child deserve a permanent time-out. Also, commercials designed to trigger the "I want that" genetic response should be skipped. What they don't see can't tempt them.
- Stay awake. Falling asleep in front of the TV or computer has been associated with sleep problems (and you don't need more of those!). Experts recommend no electronic stimulation within an hour, at least, of bedtime. And to be sure your child doesn't tune back in after the lights are turned out, remove all screens from the bedroom.

Ready to put the toys down and take a snack break? Next up, we'll share our best solutions for choosing, preparing, and storing the healthiest and safest foods available for your baby's rapidly growing body, giving him the freedom to really enjoy (and wear!) what he's eating.

Smart Solutions at a Glance

Warning Labels

- Seek out toys clearly labeled "PVC-free." If it's marked with a recycle code of 3, it likely has PVC.
- Seek out toys clearly labeled "BPA-free." A toy marked with a recycle code of 7 likely has BPA.
- Buy new and reputable brands made in the USA. If you're buying toys that have been painted, look for "nontoxic" and "lead-free" labels.
- Choose water-based markers, pens, and paints that are labeled "low-odor," "nontoxic," or stamped with the ACMI-certified product seal.
- Buy toys made of natural fibers and unfinished solid wood.

Babes in (Safe) Toyland

- Avoid small toys with pieces that can be easily yanked, snapped, or chewed off, strings that could choke, magnets that could come loose, and toys that are too loud.
- Get in the habit of giving the toys that are most frequently in play a

good wash. A natural, nontoxic dish soap with water will do, or wipe them down with an alcohol-free sanitizer.

- Keep bath toys clean and dry and the mildew away.

First Gear

- The best high chairs are made from durable, high-quality natural wood and nontoxic glue, lead-free finishes, and low-VOC paint.
- Shop for plastic tray covers that are BPA- and phthalate-free.
- Look for the JPMA certification seal.
- Shop for car seats that are free of fire retardants like PBDEs, in the lining and seat cushion, and PVC, in the plastic.
- Choose stroller sunshades with UVF protection.

An e-Motional Debate

- According to the AAP, your child can safely engage in screen time starting at age two for a limited amount of two hours a day.
- Sit and watch shows or play games together to monitor your child's screen time.
- Discuss what you're seeing and answer any questions your child might have about content. This makes for quality learning time.

Step 5

Eat Healthy and Happy

Once we became parents, we had many lightbulb moments when we looked at our own habits, and thought, "What am I doing?" From evaluating what we were using to scrub the tub to what we were putting on the dinner table, with parenthood came a sense of responsibility and an uncanny ability to look at our everyday practices through the eyes of our babies. The next time you have one of these moments, ask yourself, "What can I be doing better? Is there a safer alternative?" Our main message to you is this: There's always room for improvement, and change is possible at any time.

Because what our babies eat early on has such a dramatic and direct effect on their health and happiness today and throughout their entire lives, instilling good eating habits from day one is a practice we applaud. By making just a few adjustments to how you select and prepare foods and approach nutrition, you can achieve healthy and delicious results—and develop a child who will *choose* to eat well forever (imagine that!). In this step we'll share with you what we've learned about

- Making sense of food labels
- Reducing your exposure to harmful toxins
- Preparing and storing food in a way that's safe and easy
- Instilling healthy food habits that'll last a lifetime

Learn the Lingo

Without a doubt, nutrition is one of the most hotly debated topics on the playgrounds, at playdates, on message boards, and nearly everywhere parents hang out. What we've discovered is that eating healthy and safe is not only a smart parenting move, it's also relatively easy when you're armed with the latest information and understand the lingo.

"Gluten-free," "All-natural," "Raw," and "No GMOs"—trendy food lingo jumps out at you from nearly every supermarket aisle and food ad. But what does it all mean? Are foods with "No GMOs," for example, really healthier and safer? These products can definitely be more expensive! Are they worth paying for?

Before you look to us to provide you with that answer, understand that *we are not nutritionists.* We're really not qualified to advise you in great detail about what to eat. But again, here's what we can do: offer some sensible general recommendations based on our own experiences and what we've learned by talking at length to nutritionists, doctors, and other health-minded parents. We trust you to take it from there—do further research and make the smartest and most sensible choices for your family.

Taking your own personal tastes into account is important. While we'll be talking about terms like "organic," "natural," and "fat-free," we don't believe there's any one diet that works for every child or every family. Remember, it's all about balance and creating a sense of freedom, where your children can explore, accept, or reject, all types of foods. You can drive yourself insane (trust us, it happens!) if you try to take the "right" approach to food and nutrition, only to find that it absolutely conflicts with another. Our best advice: Learn what you can and then follow your gut. When you do that, we honestly don't think you can go wrong.

Let's start with some basic definitions.

Organic means . . .

Generally speaking, to be labeled "organic" or "organically grown," synthetic growth hormones, antibiotics, pesticides, and other unnatural ingredients were not used in the production of the food. Typically, the food is grown or raised using green and sustainable practices in balance with the natural environment, like feeding the animals organic grain and rotating crops from field to field to foster healthy soil, rather than growing the same crop in the same land space year after year. To be labeled "Certified Organic" or "USDA Organic," the food has to adhere to the toughest standards and regulations. Typically certified organic meat, poultry, and eggs have to be 100 percent produced on land that has been free of known or perceived toxic and chemical pesticides and fertilizers for at least three years prior to certification. Still, it's important to know that eating organic food isn't necessarily more nutritious than eating conventionally raised and grown food. It simply limits your exposure to pesticides, preservatives, and other potentially harmful chemicals that have no place in your baby's (or anyone in your family's) diet. Also, note that while organic foods limit your exposure, they aren't always pesticide free. Some "natural" pesticides may still be used in the growing process. If you ask us, the reduction of risk and exposure to these toxins is worth something, but what it's worth to you in terms of cost and convenience is a personal decision you have to make.

Q: **Dear Founding Fathers,**

I feel like I should know this, but what's the difference between organic and local? Is one better than the other? I'm never quite sure what to buy at my farmers' market.

A: **Dear Produce-Perplexed,**

Just because food is grown locally doesn't mean it's organic. "Local" simply means it's grown on a farm within a certain distance from your area, and fewer preservatives are used and less fuel is consumed in bringing that food to you. This is good for the planet. It also means you're supporting local farms and farmers, which, in our opinion, is good for the community. Also, it's likely that smaller, local farms aren't using harmful toxins and hormones. They usually can't afford to do so, and a personal attachment to the land often leads them to healthier farming practices. However, there is no *guarantee* that the food produced by local farms is organic and free of fertilizers, pesticides, and insecticides. You just won't know for sure unless you ask. At many farmers' markets, the person bagging up your peaches is often the very farmer who plucked them from the tree, so go ahead and ask, "Were these grown organic?" Most farmers are more than happy to explain to you their farming techniques.

According to Kevin and Keith . . .

We both love going to our local farmers' markets on Long Island. We'll wrangle the kids, pack up the strollers, and spend a morning visiting the various fresh produce booths (our kids love all the free samples) and chatting up our local farmers. It's something we look forward to each weekend throughout the spring and summer. Fresh local produce tastes so much better than what you buy in the grocery store because it was often just picked (sometimes that morning!) and hasn't traveled in refrigerated trucks across the country. Plus, the closer to the pick date you eat your food, the more nutrients your body gets to enjoy. It's a win (health) win (taste)!

Check These Out!
Jump on the Door-to-Door Farm Wagon!

Get local and organic farm-fresh produce and meat delivered to your door. Companies that deliver from a variety of local farms and organic wholesalers directly to your doorstep are sprouting up all over the country. Do an online search for "local, organic produce delivery" in your area and see what pops up. Believe it or not, buying directly from the farmer can be more affordable than shopping at your local grocery store, and it's so much yummier!

Vegan means . . .

A vegan diet refers to plant-based foods that are free of meat, dairy, eggs, and all animal based foods. It is rich in vegetables, fruits, whole grains, beans, nuts, and seeds, providing you with plenty of vitamins, minerals, antioxidants, fiber, and healthy oils while limiting calories, salt, sugar, and harmful fats. A vegan diet has also been linked to a longer life span and a reduced risk of cancer and lower rate of heart disease. Still, before you cut the meat, take some of the more extreme claims of veganism with a grain of salt. (Though limiting your sodium intake is also a good idea.) Do plenty of research and talk to your pediatrician before switching to a vegan diet for your baby who has very specific nutritional needs that might well be incompatible with such dietary limitations.

Raw means . . .

Raw, or "living," foods are uncooked and very close to their natural state, providing the body with more essential enzymes and nutrients than cooked food. (BTW, we're talking about food like raw vegetables, granola, and trail mix, not raw eggs and fish.) Raw foodies claim that eating this way gives them more energy and enhanced clarity. And while this might be true, you should be very careful about following a raw diet with your baby. As always, do your research and talk to your pediatrician before you choose a specific diet for your family.

Gluten-free means . . .

Gluten-free means a product does not contain gluten, the protein usually found in grains like wheat, barley, couscous, and bran, and in foods that toddlers often love to eat—bread, pasta, cereals, and crackers. Most people who eliminate gluten from their diet do so to treat celiac disease, an autoimmune disorder. Others go gluten-free to simply help with metabolism and digestion. A growing number of parents have discovered that their children's behavior and temperament improved once a gluten-free diet was introduced. We can't 100 percent vouch for any of these claims but if you're curious, there's no harm giving it a try. An increasing variety of gluten-free products in stores and restaurants are now available in almost every conceivable category.

Multigrain means . . .

Breads, pastas, crackers, and cereals that are multigrain have simply been made with more than *one* grain. Those grains may be the whole, heart-healthy kind, while others used to make the product are refined and stripped of minerals and nutrients. Also, many manufacturers of multigrain products add caramel and artificial coloring to make them darker and appear healthier. If you want a truly whole-grain product, look for brands labeled "100 percent whole grain" or "100 percent whole wheat."

No artificial flavors, colors, or preservatives means . . .

When a product is labeled this way, it means it is free of chemical additives used to enhance flavor, add color, or prolong the product's shelf life. Foods with preservatives and artificial colors often outlive fresh foods for months (sometimes years), and some preservatives, like butylated hydroxyanisole (BHA) and butylated hydroxytoluene (BHT), have been listed by the Department of Health and Human Services as possible carcinogens. If that isn't unappetizing enough, cheaply produced packaged foods with artificial flavors have often been designed (yes, by scientists) to taste so good, we feel the strong urge to eat more and more. So when your toddler has a meltdown because he can't have *just one more chip,* don't be too surprised! Food additives are addictive, unnatural, have no nutritional value, and are not healthy for you or your baby, so our advice is to stick to foods that have only a handful of natural ingredients.

Fat-free means . . .

Babies and toddlers under two need fat for brain development, so go whole or go home! Whole milk, yogurt, and cheese provide your baby with a big, healthy helping of the fat he needs for his rapidly growing brain. For non-dairy households, you have plenty of other healthy fat sources to choose from, including eggs, avocados, nuts, seeds, and olive oil. It's important not to eliminate fat from a growing baby's diet, and the main thing to remember about fat-free products is that just because they have no fat does not mean they aren't loaded with sugar. In fact, many manufacturers add sugar and sweeteners to fat-free products to make them tastier (especially to kids). Foods that have been stripped of their fat, like non-fat yogurt and low-calorie salad dressing, are often excessively high in the sweet stuff, along with thickeners and chemical preservatives that force your body to work overtime to digest them (and not in a fast-metabolism kind of way). The American Academy of Family Physicians warns consumers to beware of fat-free products that should really be labeled "sugar-high"!

Natural means . . .

When foods are labeled "natural," consumers often perceive this as the equivalent to organic or healthy. Not necessarily. Natural simply means that *some* of the ingredients are sourced from nature. But what about the rest? Your guess is as good as ours. "Natural" is one of those labels without a clear-cut definition and with loosey-goosey guidelines and standards that manufacturers often misuse to market their product. To know exactly what you're eating, read the ingredient list. Or look for the "Certified Naturally Grown" label, which means that farmers haven't used synthetic fertilizers, pesticides, herbicides, fungicides, or GMO crops to raise their food.

Grass-fed means . . .

The USDA's grass-fed standard for animals like cows and goats is that they must be fed only grass and forage, and have access to a pasture during the growing season. The American Grassfed Association will certify (look for the AGA logo) that cattle, bison, lambs, and goats are fed only on pasture, in addition to being raised without antibiotics and synthetic hormones, and are not confined. For other animals, like chicken and pigs, there are currently no specific certification standards for these animals being grass fed or pastured.

Free-range means . . .

Free-range poultry is generally defined as birds that don't live in cages and that spend part of their time outside, but whether that's ten minutes per month or ten hours per day is up to the farmer. The "free-range" label allows for a lot of wiggle room. Also, the USDA doesn't have a standardized or regulated definition for free-range beef or pork.

Zero trans fat means . . .

Products labeled in this way have low to no trans fats (hydrogenated and partially hydrogenated oils). Trans fats—found in fried fast foods, snack foods, and packaged baked goods like cakes and cookies—have been shown to raise cholesterol and increase the likelihood of heart disease. They've also been linked to childhood obesity and absolutely do not fall into the good-fats category. It's important to remember that just because a product is labeled "zero trans fat" doesn't mean it's healthy. It can still be full of sugar and other unnatural substances.

No artificial sweeteners means . . .

These are foods free of synthetically or chemically produced sweeteners like aspartame (Equal), saccharine (Sweet'n Low), and sucralose (Splenda). Artificial sweeteners are suspected to cause headaches, alter the nervous system, and overstimulate the brain; saccharine has even been linked to cancer. Stevia, a relative newcomer to the alternative sweetener scene, is a natural alternative made from herbs and generally regarded to be safer than the rest.

Hormone-free means . . .

"Hormone-free," "no hormones administered," or "no synthetic hormones" are general claims that imply that the farmer or manufacturer has gone *beyond* USDA regulations for conventional meat production, and that the animal was not injected with any *added* steroids or artificial hormones in its lifetime. (Just know that there is no organization certifying this claim other than the company marketing the product.) The USDA does categorically ban the use of all hormones in pork, chicken, and eggs, so these products are free of hormones whether they're labeled this way or not.

Pesticide-free means . . .

Buying "pesticide-free" is a great step toward eating better, but know that while foods with this label have been grown without synthetic pesticides, they may not be free of pesticide residues. Some organic food may be contaminated at low levels with pesticides blown in from adjacent farms or from pesticides left in the soil from past use.

No GMOs means . . .

Food products labeled "GMO-free" or "No GMOs" have not been genetically modified or engineered, although there are no federal regulations on labeling food products this way. The FDA has ruled that food that's been genetically altered is no different from "regular" food and there is currently no reliable evidence that ingredients made from GMO crops are dangerous for your baby. Still, public concern persists about the health dangers of GMO foods (corn and soybeans are the biggies), specifically pesticide exposure, antibiotic resistance, and the creation of new allergens. There is reasonable, evidence-based concern about the negative effects of GMO crops on the environment, especially the possibility that a genetically modified organism can be introduced into wild populations, leading to pesticide-resistant insects. Negative consequences to plant and wildlife biodiversity are also under investigation. The potential ripple effect of GMO crops on our ecosystem, more than any immediate health effects, is why we personally steer clear of these foods. But we encourage you to do more research and talk with other informed and trusted parents before making a decision either way.

Q: **Dear Founding Fathers,**

It seems like every food out there these days is a potential "allergen." I can't keep up! Peanuts were the first, then soy, and now wheat and GMO foods. Is identifying allergens just a current health craze, or are there certain foods I really should cut out of my child's diet?

A: **Dear Allergen-erally Confused,**

Milk, eggs, peanuts, shellfish, soy, tree nuts, and wheat. These foods are the most common allergens and yes, we agree—it *is* hard to keep up. It is true that celiac disease is on the rise and that many people who don't test positive for celiac disease find that eliminating gluten from their diets makes them feel better. But before you go gluten-free, remember that whole wheat and other whole grains like barley and oats are a tremendous source of fiber, which your growing baby needs. When it comes to foods like eggs, nuts, and fish that have a high nutritional value, our advice is to introduce a varied, moderate diet . . . and then wait. See what happens.

Allergies are real, but there is no need to avoid foods without some evidence that they're causing a bad reaction. Unless, of course, *you* have an allergy. Family history is often linked to allergies, so if you're allergic to eggs, there's a high likelihood your child will be, too, and you may want to hold off on the fried-egg sandwiches until you can confirm or dismiss this concern. Once you rule out genetics, go ahead and feed your kid an assortment of foods. Then, if certain foods negatively affect your baby's skin or behavior (the red windburn look, hives, or diarrhea are obvious red flags!), consult your pediatrician. She is your best resource for determining probable cause and how to treat food allergies. The short answer to your question: Don't worry unnecessarily about allergens. The scary stories get a lot of play online and off-line. There's not a lot of talk about the babies and children who eat everything with absolutely no problems whatsoever.

The reality is there's no scientific evidence for prominent alarmist claims such as, "Artificial sweeteners cause ADHD," or "Gluten contributes to autism," so our best advice to you is enjoy your food, don't fear it! Getting rid of *everything* potentially toxic or artificial may feel like the pure and righteous way to go, but it just isn't realistic for most families. We encourage you to determine where you personally draw the line. For your family, soda with artificial sweeteners might fall into the off-limits category (not a bad call!), whereas homemade chocolate-chip cookies may be a negotiable treat.

A Clean Plate

The way our families eat was affected by how our wives started eating during pregnancy (yes, every member of the family, including Dad, can benefit from her approach!). Every day, we eat a balanced diet of lean protein and dairy, high fiber, whole grains, and vitamin-rich fruit and veggies. We try to buy local and organic when possible. This is what we call "eating clean." That's one of the cool things about having a baby. You're pretty much forced to adopt clean solutions, and before you know it they've become lifelong habits. Since the principles of eating healthy and safe are pretty much the same during pregnancy as they ought to be at any stage in life, refer back to Step 1 for what foods can help you take steps to "clean" eating. We've included some additional considerations below.

Picking Produce

Consider: pesticides and other chemical residue

For sure, fruits and veggies help your children grow strong and thrive. When possible, we recommend including an assortment of fresh fruits and vegetables in your family's diet, and choosing produce that's low in pesticides and other chemical residues. Remember how we talked earlier about how apples, with their delicious, edible skin, are often high on the chemical-residue scale whereas kiwis are not? Lower your exposure as much as possible by choosing the safest produce and washing and scrubbing it thoroughly before eating. When fresh isn't available, frozen works just fine (so long as the ingredient listed on the back of the bag includes the produce and nothing more).

Fish

Consider: mercury and sustainability

Fish is low in fat, vitamin rich, packed with protein, and full of omega-3 fatty acids, including docosahexaenoic acid (DHA), which promotes vision and brain development and protects against heart disease and high cholesterol. Fish is a really healthy choice, but remember, it's not always the *safest* choice. The big concern with seafood is that it might heighten your exposure to methylmercury, which fish absorb and ingest as they swim and feed. Exposure to high doses of mercury may lead to language, attention, and memory problems. The FDA warns that pregnant and breast-feeding women should avoid eating bigger "top-feeder" fish like shark and swordfish, which have higher concentrations of mercury in their bodies. Minimize your risk by choosing safer types of fish and limit your intake to about twelve ounces a week (per the EPA guidelines). Refer back to Step 1 for a complete list of the healthiest fish to eat.

Milk and Dairy

Helpful Resource: Seafood Watch

Some fish are overfished (not sustainable) or farmed in a way that is harmful to the environment. An organization called Seafood Watch is a great resource for quick and easy informational guides so you know you're choosing safe and sustainable fish. Go to www.montereybayaquarium.org/seafoodwatch for their downloadable guides.

Consider: Bovine Growth Hormone (rBGH)

Milk products are high in calcium, the bone-building nutrient your growing baby needs. Dairy's also high in vitamin D, which helps the body *absorb* calcium and phosphorous. That sippy cup of milk is also full of omega-3s and fat—the good kind that fosters brain growth. So switching your baby from breast milk (or formula) to cow's milk has some big-time health benefits. As to when you make the switch is a question for your pediatrician. The AAP recommends switching at age one, while others suggest you wait longer. Some don't believe in introducing cow's milk into your child's diet at all. The debate over the benefits and risks of drinking cow's milk is one we're going to politely sit out. Remember: We're not nutritionists. What we do know is that unless you're buying organic milk or conventional milk labeled rBGH-free, you may be exposed to the recombinant bovine growth hormone that conventional farmers often give to lactating cows to boost milk production. What's the harm? Some charge that rBGH causes early puberty in kids, but the most recent scientific research does not support this claim. To date, there's no solid evidence that rBGH negatively affects people, and the FDA has determined that there is no significant difference between milk from cows treated with rBGH and non-treated cows. Still, if you want to play it safe, buy organic or look for conventional brands like Borden, Lucerne, and Wal-Mart milk that is rBGH-free. If your child has a milk allergy or if you've chosen to be a dairy-free household, know too that there are plenty of other ways for your kids to get calcium and healthy fats. Calcium-rich foods like tofu, sardines, almonds, sunflower seeds, navy beans, broccoli, and many green leafy veggies are great additions to everyone's diet. As always, discuss these issues with your pediatrician. Because, as you now know (let's say it all together now!), *we are not nutritionists*!

Q: **Dear Founding Fathers,**

I've heard that many of the toxic contaminants and pollutants we're trying to avoid can be introduced and transferred through a mother's breast milk. I understand there are a lot of things that I can do to reduce my exposure to pollutants in my own home, but I don't have a lot of control over the outside world. Is my baby better off drinking formula from a bottle? At least it's a controlled substance, right?

A: **Dear Bottle-Baffled,**

Breast milk versus formula—this is a controversial topic, and one we approach with caution. Our general attitude is do what works for *you*. Whether you decide to breast-feed or formula-feed is, in the end, a personal decision—and one you should discuss primarily with your doctor (even though you'll find friends, relatives, and perfect strangers eager to give you their advice). From the perspective of health and safety, the latest research tells us that even though outside contaminants like pesticides, mercury, and lead can be passed through a mother's breast milk, the health benefits to your baby outweigh the risks.

Breast milk contains living cells, enzymes, and antibodies, which protect your baby from a variety of infections and reduce the severity of infections when your baby does catch something. Breast milk is a nearly perfect food, naturally rich in nutrients like calcium and omega-3 fatty acids (including DHA, which stimulates brain development). There are benefits to you, too. Breast-feeding reduces your risk of breast cancer and can serve as a bonding experience between you and your child.

Meat

Consider: antibiotics and dioxins

Meat is high in protein, vitamin B12, and iron, all essential for your growing baby's health and wellness. However, meat has raised concerns because antibiotics are often given to animals to prevent disease, along with hormones to encourage rapid growth. Whether ingesting antibiotics and hormones compromises our health is not yet clear. What we do know is that overuse of antibiotics can create bacteria that are drug-resistant, making infections harder to battle. If you want to steer clear and eat only antibiotic- and hormone-free meat, buy "USDA Organic." Also know that you can find iron in places other than a sirloin steak. Check your local market or grocery store for iron-fortified cereals. There are many! Also, many nuts and seeds are packed full of iron. Pistachios are high on the list and the iron content in tofu is off the charts!

Another consideration when eating animal protein is that some fatty meats like beef may increase your risk of exposure to dioxins, like heterocyclic amines (HCAs). See our "Not So Tasty" list below to understand why dioxins are bad news. You can minimize your exposure to all three by trimming the fat, eating organic, and choosing lean proteins like poultry and seafood instead.

Kevin and Keith's NOT-SO-TASTY List

DIOXINS

Where you'll find them: Dioxins, toxic by-products that can be created in the manufacture and incineration of PVC and released into the air, hide out in soil, sneak their way into animal feed, and can end up in the fat tissue and livers of the animals we eat (beef, poultry, and fish) and in eggs and dairy. In fact, food accounts for 95 percent of human exposure to dioxins.

Why they're bad news: Dioxins can accumulate in human fat and stay in the body for many years. Studies have suggested that high dioxin levels can lead to a variety of health concerns, including birth defects, reproductive and developmental problems, and an increased risk of diabetes, immune system abnormalities, and cancer.

HETEROCYCLIC AMNES (HCAs)

Where you'll find them: In cooked and especially burned and charred muscle meats such as beef, pork, fowl, and fish. HCAs form at high-cooking temperatures, especially on grills, barbecues, fryers, and smokers.

Why they're bad news: Known carcinogens with links specifically to stomach cancer.

Gulp. That's a lot of unappetizing information to digest, but we serve it up only so you're aware of what's out there—and once again, we suggest taking a balanced approach. Not sure how? We're here to help! Let us share what we each do every day to balance nutrition and make safe food choices that give us (and our babies) the freedom to really enjoy what's on our plates.

According to Keith . . .

Our approach with our kids is far from rigid, but we have put some standards in place that we enforce every day: three balanced meals of healthy carbs, lean protein, organic fruit and veggies, and a healthy after-school snack of the kids' choosing.

After dinner they have what we call a "free pass." If they're still hungry or they want a treat, anything in the kitchen is fair game. Our reasoning? As long as they've achieved balance throughout the day and most of what they've eaten is healthy, we're cool with loosening the reins at night. Funny thing is, the kids don't really go crazy with their free passes. Believe it or not, my daughter, Skylar, will usually choose a piece of fruit or a fistful of edamame for dessert—a pretty sophisticated palate for a four-year-old. (OK, she'll sometimes go for the cotton-candy ice pop. She's a kid after all!) My son Zach on the other hand, usually takes the opportunity to snarf up a bag of chips or his favorite: chocolate-covered pretzels.

If we're so big on balanced nutrition, you may be wondering, why do we even have stuff like this in the house? Reason #1: We let our kids indulge in treats some of the time so they don't feel the urge to sneak over to a buddy's to binge on the really unhealthy stuff. In the end, we believe that a little permission goes a long way. Reason #2: (Full disclosure here) I have a sweet tooth. While the majority of the foods in the house are healthy, a top to bottom inspection of our fridge and kitchen cabinets will reveal a stockpile of goodies. My go-to treat is milk and cookies, and I'll often have them for dessert. Because I take the same balanced approach to eating as my kids, I have no guilt over this indulgence, knowing that 95 percent of my daily intake fueled and fed me in a healthy way. It's an approach I recommend to every kid and kid-at-heart.

According to Kevin . . .

In our house, we pay less attention to how much and when our kids eat and focus more on *what* they eat. Ali and I are ingredient hawks. Yeah, we're those parents in the grocery store reading the back of every package we pick up before we put it in the cart. We don't filter for everything, but you won't find us buying many packaged foods—most contain stuff that sounds like it's from another planet. Our stance is if the ingredient list is unrecognizable, unpronounceable, or *two paragraphs long*, we skip it. When you buy fresh, organic blueberries, there's only one ingredient—blueberries—and this is an ingredient we can feel really good about! We buy natural and organic whenever possible. We choose fresh over processed and avoid synthetic ingredients and artificial additives.

Also, we spend time around the dinner table talking to our kids about what they're eating, where their food comes from, and why it's so good for them. So far, we seem to have made the point successfully that when we eat artificial or "unnatural" foods, our bodies are robbed of all the natural flavors and good stuff. The truth is, kids gravitate toward healthy things like fruit if you don't introduce them to artificial sweets and salty packaged foods that once they've tasted, they start to crave. Seriously, my kids will often overlook the birthday cake, but they'll wrestle you over a bowl of fresh, sweet grapes.

We've met a lot of parents who insist that their children simply won't eat healthy foods. We then ask them, "Do *you* eat healthy foods?" Most kids eat what they are familiar with—that is, what they see Mom and Dad eating. Our kids closely model our behavior (until they're teenagers and then will of course do exactly the opposite), so if your eating habits aren't the healthiest, you can't expect theirs to be any better. If you want to change how your children eat, begin by making changes to your own eating habits and by becoming conscious of what foods you bring into your home.

Creating healthy habits is about creating *family* habits and then—have patience. Healthy eating doesn't happen overnight. It's a slow process to create habit and routine, so the earlier you start building, the better. As much as you might want to really (really!) give up on days when your child is acting particularly picky and making the icky-food face, we encourage you to hang in there.

Family Food Fun

Once you're feeling good about the foods you've carefully selected for your family, it's time to get cooking! Are you a make-it-from-scratch or a ready-to-serve kind of parent? Either way, we don't judge you. We're believers in doing whatever works for you and your family, and what we've discovered is that what works in the Schwartz household doesn't necessarily work for the Garbers.

Check These Out!

Healthy Kid Snacks

The way we see it, snacks are mini meals, so it's important they're packed full of nutrition. Try offering these tasty and healthy snacks to your kids once or twice a day.

-Cut-up apple with nut butter
-Hummus and snap peas
-String beans and cheese cubes
-Carrot-zucchini bread
-Guacamole with wholegrain pita chips
-Edamame
-Turkey jerky
-Bean and cheese quesadillas
-Mini meatloaves and quiches (made in muffin pans)
-Homemade trail mix: dried fruit, unsalted nuts, and dry cereal
-Yogurt or kefir fruit smoothie
-Egg salad on whole-grain bread

According to Keith . . .

Check This Out!

Baby Food On-the-Go

- Earth's Best (www.earthsbest.com)
- GoGo squeeZ (www.gogosqueez.com)
- Happy Family Organic Superfoods (happyfamilybrands.com)
- Plum Organics (www.plumorganics.com)

When Zach was born, Nicole and I were determined that once he started on solid foods, we'd make everything from scratch. We bought all the equipment, gadgets, and books. We were both super-motivated and excited to use it all—and we did it! For about a month. Then one day we looked at each other and knew we were done. We were both juggling new parenthood and full-time jobs, and running an organic baby food factory was just too much. If you can make it work, we applaud you. If you find the DIY approach overwhelming, don't worry: There are many amazing organic and healthy on-the-go and ready-to-eat options out there. We especially love the baby food pouches that kids and even some babies can hold themselves.

According to Kevin . . .

I'm not saying that Ali and I are the world's best parents (and clearly no one is a better dad than Keith!), but from the get-go, both Ali and I have been committed to doing it ourselves, preparing all the food that goes into our babies' bellies. I'm talking homemade baby food purees of avocado and peas and sweet potato and prune; and once they were six months old or so, introducing solids like chicken with veggies we'd make in the slow cooker. Making it all yourself can be messy and time-consuming, but for us it has always felt worth it. As parents, making your own food is one of the most direct and effective actions you can take to feel confident that what's introduced into your children's bodies is healthy and safe.

Over the years, we must have tried every gadget out there to perfect our natural food-prep techniques and get it right and honestly, all you really need is a simple, reliable tool to chop, grind, or purée your baby's food. While there are many sleek and snazzy all-in-one gadgets out there (that you might—*hint, hint*—consider adding to your baby shower registry), you can save yourself some money by relying on this time-tested, inexpensive, portable, nonelectric gadget: the fork. Yeah. Just a plain old fork. This most basic of kitchen equipment does a great job mashing up food. All you need is a little patience.

Clean and safe: top of mind, all the time

Food prep goes hand in hand with food safety, so before you handle any food with those squeaky-clean hands of yours, you'll want to create a clean and safe space to prepare your special of the day. This is easy-peasy work but you do need to be vigilant—wipe your countertops clean, and scrub your cutting boards, dishes, and utensils with hot soapy water *every time.* Be sure your sponges, brushes, and dish wands have been recently sanitized (or replaced if they're looking all ragged or generally gunky). Oh, and don't forget those kitschy kitchen towels your sister-in-law gave you. Just because they came from Anthropologie doesn't mean they don't get dirty!

Along with keeping a clean kitchen, be sure that the food you're about to prepare has been thoroughly washed and cleaned. Remember, dark leafy greens like kale, cabbage, and spinach make a great hideout for residual pesticides used in the growing process, especially on their outer leaves. Unless you buy organic or grow everything yourself, they'll need a good rinsing before they're safe to eat. Go back to Step 1 for a list of the safest fruits and vegetables on the market and the smartest solutions for reducing your exposure to pesticides. Finally, dedicate a separate prep area for fresh produce and another one for handling raw meat and poultry to reduce the risk of exposure to bacteria such as Salmonella and E coli. They can migrate from raw meat into your vegetables and cause infection.

Q: **Dear Founding Fathers,**

Wooden or plastic cutting boards? Plastic is certainly lighter, cheaper, and easier to clean, but I've recently read reports that wood might actually be healthier and safer. Which do you prefer?

A: **Dear Stumped Over Wood,**

We used to think non-porous plastic that can be easily thrown into a sanitizing dishwasher was cleaner and therefore safer, but as far as minimizing infectious bacteria goes, wood may be the better choice. A plastic cutting board quickly becomes nicked by knives and utensils and over time those cuts and crevices become nearly impossible to clean, even in a hot dishwasher, and this is exactly where bacteria like to hide out. Wooden boards, on the other hand, may actually trap bacteria in its deep grooves where they die after a few hours as the wood dries. A creepy case of bacteria buried alive! In our homes, we use both wood and plastic boards for different aspects of food preparation and take a commonsense, baby-safe approach: avoid cross-contamination by having at least two cutting boards, one designated for fresh produce and the other for cutting raw meat, poultry, and fish. After every use (make a pledge of allegiance, now!), scrub them good and clean with hot soapy water, and replace your cutting boards every couple of years.

Food prep is fairly simple in the first six months of your baby's life when the majority of her foods consist of smashed-up fruits and veggies along with a whole-grain, iron-fortified cereal that doesn't require much more than a quick stir. But once your baby starts eating real solids and you find yourself cooking again, there are hot items to be aware of. One of the biggies is PFOA.

Kevin and Keith's
HOT list

PERFLUOROOCTANOIC ACID (PFOA)

Where you'll find it: A synthetic chemical compound found in nonstick cookware like Teflon and some waterproof, breathable clothing.

Why it's bad news: PFOA makes cooking and cleanup easy (and what parent doesn't love that?), but when nonstick pans get super hot—over 500° F (not too likely, but it can happen)—it breaks apart and emits perfluorooctanoic acid (PFOA), a man-made chemical that's a suspected carcinogen that can build up in the bloodstream and linger for years. PFOA blood levels in humans may be linked with higher-than-normal cholesterol levels, thyroid disease, reduced fertility, and low birth weight in babies. As always, we prefer a baby-safe approach, so you might consider restocking your kitchen with pots and pans made with stainless steel or cast iron instead.

Serve it up!

You've prepared a healthy meal in a safe and clean kitchen, but before you serve that delicious meal to your wailing baby or your fitful toddler, there's one more thing to consider—what do you serve it on? Seems pretty simple, but we'll say it anyway: use plates, cups, bottles and utensils that are clearly labeled "non-toxic." Since most tableware for kids is made out of unbreakable and easy-to-wash plastic, let's review good versus not-so-good plastics.

Plastics with BPA and PVC can leach harmful chemicals into your food, especially when that leftover plate of spaghetti is heated up, so choose safe plastics that are clearly labeled "BPA-free" and "PVC-free" or that are marked with a recycling code of 1, 2, 4, and 5. Generally, soft or cloudy-colored plastic doesn't contain BPA. If it's not clearly labeled, look for plastics including polyaminc, polypropylene, and polyethylene. In the chemical world, these are the good guys. If you have any concerns about that plastic cup, plate, or bottle in your hands, put it down and opt for dishware made from safe materials like glass, ceramic, or stainless steel.

So now that your child has finished his meal (i.e. thrown it all over the floor), what do you do with the—assuming there are any—leftovers? Wrap them in plastic and stick them in the fridge? Not so fast. Did you know that many cling wraps contain PVC, which can leach phthalates? Keep the cling wrap from coming into direct contact with your food. Opt for wrapping food in waxed paper or aluminum foil, or store leftovers in glass instead. We like refrigerating and freezing extra portions of food in stackable ice cube trays. It's a super manageable storage technique and a space saver!

Q: Dear Founding Fathers,

I keep hearing that I should never heat food in plastic. So my question is, does this go for "safe"

Check This Out!

Natural Dishware

GREEN SPROUTS (www.iplaybabywear.com)

Green Sprouts makes bottles, cups, dishes, and cutlery that are PVC-free, BPA-free and made from non-petroleum materials. Green Sprouts products undergo extensive testing and conform to U.S. ASTM, FDA, and CPSC standards.

MODERN-TWIST (modern-twist.com)

Modern-twist makes 100 percent all-natural silicone place mats and bibs for kids. Recyclable and reusable. Modern-twist products are free of BPA, lead, latex, phthalates, and other harsh chemicals, and they leave a minimal carbon footprint.

PRESERVE (www.preserveproducts.com)

Preserve dishes are made in the USA from recycled materials and are BPA- and PVC-free.

plastics as well? Should I keep those out of the microwave, too?

BAMBU
(www.bambuhome.com)
Bambu makes kids dishware and utensils from bamboo. They create safe products from chemical-free sources, and their products are manufactured without glue or lacquers that can leach into your food.

A: **Dear Heated Over Microwaves,**
If you're using tableware that's clearly labeled "nontoxic," "BPA-free," "PCV-free," or has a recycling code of 1, 2, 4, or 5, you can put it into the microwave and feel pretty confident that harmful chemicals are not seeping into your food. Still—to remove any doubt—we recommend heating and reheating food in glass and covering it with a cloth or paper napkin. Cling wrap, which is plastic, can leach phthalates into your food, especially as it's heated. Plus, if you've put cling wrap in the microwave you know how much clingier it gets when you try to remove it. Talk about a hot mess!

As your baby grows and becomes more curious about what you're doing in the kitchen, consider inviting him to cook alongside you. We love step stools and kitchen helpers, like the Little Partners Learning Tower, that safely bring your toddler up to counter level where she can easily participate in the action. Give him his own mixing bowl, a few measuring spoons, a wooden spoon—everything he needs to create a culinary master mess! Cut up an assortment of foods and let him explore different textures, shapes, colors, and tastes. Not only is food prep the perfect time to school your kids on the benefits of healthy foods and nutritional eating, it's a fun way to include and engage your children. It encourages them to take part in the meal and helps to connect them to the food they're about to eat.

But before your budding chef turns your kitchen upside down, consider these smart solutions.

SMART SOLUTIONS:
Kitchen Safety for Little Cooks

- Access denied! Secure baby-unsafe areas such as the cellar stairs with safety gates, install safety latches on cabinets with heavy pots and on drawers with sharp knives, and cover hot stove tops with knob covers.
- Stash the trash. Keep icky trash cans hidden away or use cans with child-proof lids.
- A drawer of his own. Keep one easy-to-reach cupboard or drawer unlocked and filled with fun, child-safe cookware to play with, like wooden spoons, a mini colander, rolling pin, and plastic measuring cups. When your baby has his own drawer, he's less interested in the place you don't want him to get into!

Mealtime

So you've gone to all this trouble to create a child-friendly kitchen. You invite your little one to share in the preparation of the family meal. You give her an assortment of kitchen gadgets and ingredients to play with and you gently stress the importance of healthy eating and yet—be prepared. In no way is this a guarantee that she'll eat what's served at the table.

According to Kevin . . .

This happens to every parent—your kid reaches a certain age and his favorite expression becomes "Why? Why? Why?" I'm a healthy eater, but I admit, I'm also kind of picky, so when Ali and I try to tempt our son Tyler into trying something new, he'll say, "Why isn't Daddy trying it?" That's when Ali will glance (ever so lovingly) in my direction and say, "Yes, Daddy, why *aren't* you trying it?" Busted! If I want my kids to eat their veggies, then I have to eat mine, too. With certain foods I've gotta take one for the team, put on my best "Mmmmmmm, yummy" grin and dig in. But Tyler knows me well. He can tell when I'm faking it, and he finds it hilarious to watch me gag down a forkful of cauliflower (not my favorite). After he's done laughing I can usually get him to take at least one bite, and next time, I can probably coax him to take two, maybe three. Developing a taste for some foods takes time, and everyone has their personal preferences. Just remember that tastes change, so we recommend reintroducing kids to foods they may have hated last month. We're not big on force-feeding and making meals into unhappy moments, but we're firm about asking our kids to try everything and eat a healthy mix of foods.

Another tactic we often use is the "taste test game." We put two foods that are similar in size and texture, like cauliflower and broccoli, on the table. I'll close my eyes and let Tyler feed me and I have to guess which is which, and then it's my turn. Before he realizes it—because he's still laughing from watching me suffer through the cauliflower—Tyler has eaten several new foods without the resistance and fear that can often go along with trying something unfamiliar.

We're both big fans of the family meal. Preparing meals at home and sitting down together at least once a day is integral to both of the Schwartz and Garber lifestyles. Did you know that eating dinner as a family less than five times a week *doubles* a preschooler's risk of obesity? Not only are regular meals together a healthy habit, they are a great chance for parents to lead by example. At times it sure doesn't feel like it, but parents really can be persuasive (we promise!). When our kids see us enjoying healthy and natural foods, they're more willing to try them.

Little known fact: It takes a child up to fifteen tries before she'll accept a new food as familiar. This means: Don't give up! Your child's taste buds are changing every day. What she loves on Monday might make her gag on Friday, and vice versa. If you have a picky eater, continue to *offer*—not guilt, force, or bribe (as tempting as it may be)—an assortment of wholesome foods. Do your best to broaden her menu, and don't be surprised if she takes one bite and spits out your goat cheese and spinach lasagna. It happens! Just reintroduce it in a few weeks. It also doesn't hurt to get creative and present it in a different form (spinach and goat cheese frittata, anyone?). At some point, your kids will likely come around. Many parents can become discouraged by their children's fickle tastes and before they realize it, they become short-order cooks in their own kitchens. Hey, you're running a household, not a restaurant!

According to Keith . . .

No kids' menus in our home. At mealtime, we all eat the same thing (or at least, we're all *served* the same thing). If Zach or Skylar chooses not to touch what we've prepared that night, we don't make a huge deal out of it because we know it'll be returning to the table, and probably very soon. Getting into a battle over food is no fun. So if one of them makes the icky-food face, we sit back—try to relax—and ask that they at least give it a try.

From early on, Nicole and I have delivered a consistent message: In our house we eat healthy food because it makes us feel good. It helps our brains and bodies work better. Kids understand *smarter, faster,* and *stronger.* When we first introduced spinach to Zach, he made a face. He said, "Looks weird, no way I'm eating that." But when I explained to him that spinach builds muscles and will help him grow strong, he gobbled it all up. When I was a kid my mom told me carrots helped me see in the dark and that worked, too!

Eating out

Cooking takes time, and if you're like most parents, you don't have much to spare. Make life easy and plan for meals ahead of time. Plot out your menu for a full week and shop for everything you'll need in one go. When you have everything on hand, you're guaranteed a healthy meal—and you're not running to the store during an already hectic day. Consider cooking more than one meal at a time so you don't have to prepare a fresh meal seven days a week. Cook large portions and freeze the leftovers for another night.

Do all this, and still . . .

There are going to be nights when you just want to eat out or order in. We say go for it! Take a night off. You deserve it! When it comes to eating out, our philosophy is simple: how our family eats outside the home is just an extension of how we eat inside the home. We take our safe and healthy habits with us wherever we go, and we just love these parent-tested smart solutions for making safe and healthy choices when eating out.

SMART SOLUTIONS:

Eating Out Doesn't Mean Giving Up!

- Avoid fast food. Research tells us that, on average, a child will consume nearly two hundred calories more when eating fast food rather than a home-cooked meal.
- Avoid fried food. Choose grilled or baked instead. Less fat, more nutritional value.
- Choose water or milk over soda or juice. Less sugar, fewer meltdowns.
- Snack first. If your child has eaten a nutritious snack *before* leaving the house, he is less likely to throw an "I'm starving" tantrum in the middle of the restaurant.
- Seek out a healthy kids' menu. A lot of restaurants now offer more than grilled cheese, chicken strips, and fries. They've finally caught on—kids like a variety of healthy foods, too!
- Bring food from home. Not sure what the options will be? Don't want your kids dining exclusively on dinner rolls? Pack a few healthy choices from your kitchen to bring along.
- Seek local and fresh. Locally owned restaurants that serve fresh, organic food will provide you with the greatest number of healthy options.
- Order off the menu. You were hoping to order a bean, cheese, and veggie quesadilla, but it's not on the menu. No problem. Order it anyway. If they have the raw ingredients, trust us—they can make it.

- Healthy sides. Order a side of fruit or veggies instead of fries or chips.
- Avoid family-style. Yes, you're a family, but your child's little belly doesn't need a huge platter of food. She just can't stomach it! "All you can eat" isn't a great idea for adults *or* kids.
- Don't force kids to finish. Everyone at the table is digging in, but your daughter would rather build a card house with sugar packets than finish her meal. Let it go. Yes, you just spent good money on that plate of cheese ravioli but encouraging your child to eat *every last one* whether or not she's hungry is not a healthy habit.
- When the food starts flying, the meal is over.

According to Keith . . .

The thing about eating outside the home is that you have a whole lot less control over your options and how the food's prepared. Is the kitchen clean? How healthy is the food? Where did it come from? If you let your mind run wild (or watch too many episodes of *Kitchen Nightmares*), you can lose your appetite before you even place your order.

I like a restaurant with an open kitchen so I can see what's going on behind the line. When I order take-out for Nicole and the kids, it's from restaurants I've been to many times and that I know are healthy and clean. We have a tradition of ordering take-out Thai on Sunday nights. We always get it from the same place that makes the most amazing spring rolls. It's a fun wrap-up (pun intended!)

to the weekend. It gives Nicole and me a break from kitchen duty, and the kids love it.

Say Aahhh!

One more thing to remember after meals . . . brush teeth! As soon as your kids have them, get brushing. The American Academy of Pediatrics and American Dental Association recommend brushing teeth at least twice a day and a first visit to the dentist at age one.

When it comes to cleaning your baby's tiny teeth and gums it's all about what's *not* going into their bodies. Fluoride has long been added to toothpaste to kill bacteria and prevent tooth decay, but the AAP advises that during the early "training phase" (until about age three, when they learn to spit it all out) kids shouldn't be around fluoride. What's the risk? It depends on whom you ask. The U.S. Centers for Disease Control (CDC) warns that one side effect from swallowing too much fluoride (whether accidentally or purposefully) is dental fluorosis, in which the tooth enamel becomes discolored. While this is generally considered a cosmetic concern and not all that harmful, there are still those who maintain that fluoride shouldn't be ingested by any child; they argue that it's a toxic chemical akin to a disinfectant. Others believe that fluoride is perfectly safe.

We take a stand somewhere in the middle. When we developed our training-phase toothpaste, we decided to take a less-is-more approach. Because fluoride isn't an essential nutrient, and because children under the age of two aren't so good at gargling and spitting (and they will be losing their baby teeth anyway), we left it out. We believe you can naturally remove plaque and gently clean your baby's teeth and gums without introducing a risk of swallowing fluoride. While we think a minimal amount of fluoride in drinking water is probably safe, eating toothpaste loaded with it—not so much.

According to Keith . . .

In our house, brushing teeth is like washing hands. It's just something we *do.* For as long as Zach and Skylar can remember, they've started their day the same way—they wake up, walk into the bathroom, wash hands, and brush teeth. It's what Daddy does. It's what Mommy does. Thus, it's what they do. (Even on the weekends, I hear them shuffling down the hall toward the bathroom as soon as they wake up. It's pretty impressive, if I do say so myself!) As we've done with hand washing, Nicole and I have instilled the habit in our kids by making it fun and by clearly explaining the benefits: Healthy teeth make beautiful smiles!

Are you full of food and nutritional info? Let's move on! Next, we'll cover everything from bathing, grooming, cleaning up after, and playing with your fur babies in a way that keeps them and everyone else in your house healthy and safe.

Smart Solutions at a Glance

Learn the Lingo

- Eating safe and healthy is relatively easy when you're armed with the right information and have a basic understanding of terms like "gluten-free," "all-natural," "raw," "organic," and "no preservatives."

A Clean Plate

- Strive to eat a balance of lean protein and dairy; high fiber, whole grains; and vitamin-rich fruits and veggies. Buy local and choose organic when possible. Avoid synthetic ingredients and artificial additives.
- When picking produce, consider pesticides and other chemical residues.
- When choosing fish, think about mercury and sustainability.
- When buying milk and dairy, consider the effects of rBGH.
- When selecting meat, think about antibiotics and dioxins.

Food Prep & Play

- Use pots and pans, plates, cups, bottles, and utensils that are clearly labeled "nontoxic," "PFOA-free," "BPA-free," and "PVC-free."

- Opt for wrapping food in waxed paper or aluminum foil, or store leftovers in glass instead.
- In the kitchen, rcstrict access to child-unsafe areas: secure the cellar stairs with safety gates, pantries with door locks, and stove tops with knob covers.
- Keep one cupboard unlocked and filled with lightweight, child-safe items.

Mealtime

- If you want to change how your children eat, begin by making changes to your own eating habits.
- Developing a taste for some foods takes time. Continue to reintroduce your children to a variety of foods.
- Regular meals together are a healthy habit and a great chance for parents to lead by example.
- Consider brushing your child's teeth with a fluoride-free toothpaste during the "training phase" (until about age three, when she learns to spit it all out).

Step 6

Your Fur Babies Matter, Too

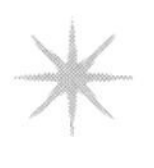

Let's just admit it: Most of us with both pets and babies are guilty of neglect. Not of our babies. Of our firstborn . . . our pets! Since you brought that tiny, new human home from the hospital, how much attention has your four-legged baby gotten? Has he taken a permanent spot in the corner or under a table? Have you ever suddenly realized you skipped a meal or left the litter unchanged? Don't beat yourself up. We've been there. We were pet guys before we became dads to human babies. And here's the good news: By taking steps to make your home healthier and safer for your baby, you've simultaneously made it a better place for your pets.

If you think about it, you'll realize our babies and pets have a lot in common. They're both low-lying creatures with fragile immune systems, and they like to roll around on the floor, licking and eating everything in sight. If it hits the ground it's theirs! Creating a home environment where your baby can play, grow, and thrive, and switching to products and solutions that are cleaner and safer, means your pets are benefitting as well. (That should relieve some of your guilt, right?)

Having a pet is very much like having a baby. How well you tend to your baby's needs has a direct impact on the health and safety of your pets. And it works the other way around, too. How well you take care of your pet's needs influences the health and safety of your child. So: safe for baby = safe for pet. In this step we'll share with you what we've learned about

- The best grooming practices for tackling allergens
- Making the best of a buggy situation
- Minimizing mess with a minimum of fuss
- Pet-proofing your home
- How both your babies can play together safely

Clean and Coiffed

Like our babies', our dogs' and cats' skin can be highly sensitive, making it susceptible to moisture loss and drying, and you know what comes next—

shedding! Not only does shedding make your floors a hairy mess, but it also spreads dander, which is potentially bad news for your baby because pet dander ranks high on the allergen list. Pet fur easily traps pollen, dust, and mold, as well as anything else your pets runs into or rolls around in, and an allergic reaction in your baby can show up in a number of different ways, including itchy, watery eyes, congestion, sneezing, runny nose, and wheezing. Eczema, asthma, rashes, and hives are also clues that your baby or child might be having an allergic reaction to your pet. Now, before you start thinking you need to find another home for your best buddy, know that most children born into a home with a dog or cat are at a low risk of developing asthma or allergies. Still, it's a smart idea to eliminate any and all triggers. Since the symptoms of pet allergies are a lot like a common cold, notice if they're year-round as opposed to seasonal. That runny nose that just won't quit is a strong indicator your child has developed a pet allergy.

While we can't stop our pets from shedding, we can significantly limit how much and how frequently they shed, and one of the quickest and easiest ways to do this is by regularly getting your pet into the bath (although, as you probably well know, some animals are more tolerant of bathing than others). When it comes to keeping your pets clean we believe in being just as selective when choosing products as you are with your baby. Many pet shampoos contain parabens, sulfates, phthalates, alcohol, and synthetic fragrances—the same toxic ingredients you want to keep away from your baby. When they're applied to your pet's coat and come in contact with his skin, the results aren't much better. For this reason, we recommend choosing pet shampoos and conditioners that are pH-balanced and made with plant-based ingredients like tea-tree oil, aloe, and vitamin E, and omega-3 fatty acids that both moisturize fur and work wonders at keeping the skin and coat healthy and flake-free.

Q: Dear Founding Fathers,

My dog doesn't get visibly dirty so I just bathe her when she starts to smell, which isn't very often. Is this good enough? I never know how often I should bathe my dog. Help!

A: Dear Bath-Befuddled,

It depends on the time of year. If it's wintertime, bathing once a month is probably enough, but if we're talking summer, we're sorry to say . . . often! Since the hotter months cause our animals to shed more, we recommend bathing your dog once a week. In addition to a regular bathing schedule, spend a few minutes a day brushing your dog. This might seem like a lot, but in our opinion (and we think your pets would agree), you can't brush your dog or cat too much. Regular brushing, like bathing, cuts down on the shedding, dander, and dust balls your pet is spreading around the house, and it can also be a wonderful bonding time. Your pets love how it feels and are grateful for the extra TLC.

Once you switch to a natural shampoo that won't dry the skin and create more dander, your next step is to get into a bathing habit of lather, quick rinse, and . . . *rinse, rinse, rinse!* Depending on your dog and the heaviness of her coat, a thorough rinsing can be a serious undertaking. We've been there! We know it's a whole lot easier getting the shampoo on than it is rinsing it off. Not only are you dealing with a lot of sudsy wet hair or fur, most dogs don't like sitting still, and if you give her the chance, you'll have a slippery wet ball running wild in your house.

But here's why you have to rinse: Residual shampoo and conditioner that get trapped in the coat or dry on the skin can become an irritation and then your pup is back to where she started—more shedding, more dander, more dust balls on the floor and allergens in the air. Not to mention that when your children pet and love on the family dog, they, too, come into contact with that residual soap, and who knows what kind of reaction they'll have. So repeat after us—rinse, rinse, rinse!

According to Kevin . . .

I know this might sound sneaky, but a great way to teach your kids responsibility at an early age is to put them to work as a groomer. (*Shhhhh*—they don't think they're doing "work.") Both my boys love bathing Tucker. They think it's the most fun in the world and they've been happily helping me on the grooming front since they were both just a few years old. On Saturdays, as soon as we return from the dog park, we all head to the bath. Tyler lathers Tucker, Ryan rinses him, and I man the shower curtain. I'm pretty good at anticipating the moment right before Tucker is going to shake (about nine shakes a bath) and spray suds and water all over the place. That's when I yell, "Clear the decks!!" and pull the curtain shut. My success rate is around 50 percent. By the time we're done, we're soaked, but Tucker's clean and the kids have had a blast.

By the way, in case I'm not the only human on the planet who didn't know this, cats don't need to be bathed. The first—and last—time I dropped our cat in the tub, I got the mother of all death stares and she wouldn't come near me for a week. Turns out cats are more than capable of cleaning themselves. Who knew?

What a lot of pet-parents don't realize is that shedding is cyclical, meaning it shouldn't be year-round. In the hot summer and dry winter months expect to see your pets shed a lot of hair, but throughout the rest of the year they shouldn't generally shed. If your pet is shedding every month, something's not quite right. So take a close look. The condition of your pet's skin and coat can tell you a lot about his health. Does your pet have dry and brittle hair? Is your dog's coat dull? Does your kitty itch and shed often? If the answer is yes, consider what your pet is coming into contact with, directly or indirectly. Remember, excess shedding isn't just a sign that something is off with your pet; it creates a potentially unsafe environment for your baby.

If you're bathing your dog once a week with a nontoxic, natural, and plant-based shampoo and conditioner and he's *still* shedding and itching, has dry and broken hair, or there's evidence of a skin irritation or an allergic reaction, it's time to consider what else you're using on or around your pet that may be irritating him. Go back to Step 2 and take an inventory. What is your animal coming into contact with inside the home?

As you know by now, many traditional household cleaning products cut through dirt and grime at the expense of our babies'—and pets'—health and safety. So think hard—is your pet being exposed to any chemically treated surfaces inside the home? Take a mental walk around your living space with a dog's-eye view. What are you using to clean the floors and surfaces in the living room and the kitchen that your pets might be rolling around and playing on? In the bathroom, are you using anything that may be leaving behind a toxic residue? What type of laundry detergent are you using to wash the dog or cat bed? Look out for potentially irritating chemicals or synthetic ingredients. Finally, consider your pets' favorite hideouts and hangouts—the front porch, garage, basement, and attic. Is there anything potentially toxic in any of these places that your pet may be bumping into, licking, or inhaling? Believe it or not, your pets' skin issues and breathing problems often go away when you simply change the products you use on the floors where your animals sleep and on the surfaces they eat from. It's a pretty quick and easy solution, and it makes a big impact.

According to Kevin . . .

I totally remember that "Aha!" moment when I first realized the risk of using cleaning products made with harmful chemicals around the house. It was in 2001 and my Labrador puppy (my first baby), Tucker, started getting these weird, irritated hot spots under his chin. My wife and I couldn't figure out what they were or where they came from, so we took him to the vet. She asked, "What's he coming into contact with?" and told us to start watching his habits.

That night Ali and I took our regular spots on the couch to watch some mindless TV (a pre-kids luxury!). Tucker, as usual, squeezed between us on the couch and rested his chin on our glass coffee table. That's when it hit us. I honestly think we both said it out loud . . . "The coffee table!" The next morning, I called our vet and she asked me, "What are you using to clean the table?"

"Uh . . . the typical 'Blue Stuff'!"

Tucker was having an allergic reaction to our glass cleaner. I started doing my homework and discovered that the main ingredient in most glass cleaners is ammonia, which is highly toxic. According to our vet, an animal's skin and coat is extremely susceptible to harsh chemicals. She suggested we stop using our go-to glass cleaner for a month. "See what happens." It was crazy how fast we saw a change. In less than a month, Tucker's hot spots completely went away. There was no denying that the ammonia in the product had been a major irritant to Tucker's skin.

You're probably not surprised to learn that your pet is as vulnerable as your baby. Because of their weak immune system, when they lick a floor that's been recently mopped with ammonia or bleach, they have a hard time recovering from ingesting the toxins. As a result, they can easily become irritated and sick, so in addition to cleaning up your house for your baby's sake, do everything you can to minimize your pet's exposure to toxic chemicals and pollutants that can make a mess of your pet's skin, coat, and overall health and happiness.

A Buggy Situation

We love our pets, but they can create a buggy situation! Even the cleanest cats and dogs can attract pests like the household dust mite, which feeds on pet dander. (Not to mention the shedding of human skin. But let's not go there, OK?) Besides being doggone gross, the problem with mites is that, like dander, they pose a potential health risk; their droppings are a common trigger for allergies and asthma, especially in babies and children—from sneezing and wheezing to watery eyes, breathing problems, and respiratory distress. And while you can't totally eliminate dust mites (in most homes they've taken up permanent residence), the easiest way to control them is to give them less to live on. Cut off their food supply by keeping your pets and house clean!

By adopting the smart solutions below, you can keep pet dander under control, fight dust mites, *and* minimize most pet allergens.

SMART SOLUTIONS:
Controlling Allergens

- Forbidden furniture. Nothing traps animal dander like the nooks and crannies of your furniture. If denying your dog or cat his favorite napping chair feels cruel, try covering it with a blanket or throw that you can remove and wash easily.
- Vacuum like you mean it. Dander and dust mites survive well in carpet-

ing and rugs. If you haven't already, invest in vacuum with a HEPA (high-energy particulate air) filter, which will trap not only animal dander but also dust-mite droppings. It's a safe idea to vacuum when your toddler is out of the room. Did you know it takes nearly two hours for allergens stirred up by vacuum cleaning to settle back down?

- Dust diligence. Dust where dander likes to collect and hang out—blinds and textured curtains are the worst offenders. Remember to avoid scattering dust with a feather brush. Instead, wipe down surfaces with a damp cloth.
- Air care. Since dust, dander, and airborne animal allergens can be circulated by your home's central heating and air-conditioning systems, consider purchasing a home air purifier to prevent the recirculation of bad air that might cause allergies.
- Bed and pillows and mites, oh my! Dust mites thrive and can survive for a long time in these cozy areas where skin flakes and pet dander collect. Make sure to wash your child's bedding frequently.
- Bedroom boundaries. Make your child's bedroom a pet-free zone, at least while they're very young, or until you can determine whether or not your child has a pet allergy. Pets in the bed may be cute, but it's not healthy or safe.
- Get tough on stuffed. Limit your baby's stuffed buddies to one or two, and launder them once a week in water that is at least 140° F.

Flea-free

The truth is that you can be extra vigilant about creating a clean indoor space, but unless your pet is exclusively an inside dweller, it's only a matter of time before something pesky rides into your home on the backside of your favorite four-legged friend. And what are the most common of all cat and dog infestations? Fleas!

Prevention is key when it comes to fleas, because once those little buggers lay eggs and spread throughout your house, they can be tough to eliminate. Did you know that the common cat flea will not only take residence in her fur, but also attack nearby dogs and other animals? Nasty! Infants are vulnerable to developing an allergic rash when bitten, and older children who love to nuzzle their favorite furry friends are at an increased risk of suffering from itchy bites. By keeping your pets regularly washed and brushed, by vacuuming regularly and maintaining a clean home, you're doing almost everything you can to prevent it from becoming a flea-bag motel.

By now you know we love the natural approach. And while it's true that a dog bed filled with cedar chips can repel fleas, and many nontoxic flea collars scented with herbs like citronella, rosemary, and lemongrass can drive fleas away, when it comes to combating fleas, the natural solutions aren't always effective. Therefore, our best advice is to consult your vet about flea prevention and then take a *minimalist* approach. Use chemicals sparingly. Pills that leave no chemical residue on your pet's coat are our favorite option. Topical medications like Comfortis, Trifexis, Frontline, Advantage, Revolution, or Vectra are effective, too, but they can be unsafe for babies when touched. Since it can be hard keeping little hands off the family pet, use them only as needed. Then enforce a "no-petting" rule until the medication has dried and your furry companion is once again safe to snuggle.

Q: **Dear Founding Fathers,**

We're so beyond prevention. We have a full-blown flea infestation. Is the flea bomb safe?

A: **Dear Flea Fighters,**

As you can probably guess, we're not big fans of bombing anything. While a flea bomb might be effective, it's toxic! Avoid it if possible. Insecticide residue from a flea bomb can collect on upholstery, rugs, carpeting, and stuffed animals. It also contaminates the air. But it sounds like the fleas have gotten comfortable, and we appreciate your itching desire to take action, especially if you have a newborn in the house. We say, call in the pros! A pest control specialist can likely help you handle the situation without dropping a bomb. Choose a company that uses non-chemical treatments, and in the future, do everything you can to prevent fleas from dropping in unannounced.

On to another mess. Yeah . . . that kind. Pet allergies aren't caused only by dander and dust mites, but also from coming into contact with our pets' droppings. If you have a cat, consult your obstetrician early on in your pregnancy. She'll likely tell you that pregnant women should avoid handling kitty litter for the duration of the pregnancy, as first-term babies are especially at risk for contracting a virus called toxoplasmosis, which you can get by handling cat litter, the litter box, or the box liner. Dads, that means roll up your sleeves and grab the scooper!

Most cats are good at thinking inside the box—the litter box that is—but accidents will happen. When they do, we encourage you to skip the highly fragranced chemical cleaners. For pets and children, floors are a place to play, nap, and crawl around—they're no place for harsh and toxic fresheners. When accidents and odors happen, get them gone with nontoxic solutions that fight tough pet stains and the stinkiest of smells—naturally.

SMART SOLUTIONS:
Minimize the Mess

- Do not rub. To remove a pet urine stain, dampen a rag with water and dab or blot it up before it soaks into your furniture. Rubbing will set the stain.
- Counter the smell. Blot the "accident" site with a natural, nontoxic stain and odor remover derived from plants. Choose one with a natural scent like lemon verbena or tangerine to counter unwanted animal smells.
- Control the stink. To eliminate deep-down odors, sprinkle baking soda on the spot and leave overnight, then vacuum. Avoid using a steamer to clean pet stains or a hair dryer to dry them. Heat causes stains and odors to set, making them virtually impossible to remove.

- Re-soil alert! Ever notice how ammonia smells a lot like cat pee? Well, it does to your cat, too. Steer clear of using products containing ammonia to clean up an "accident" because your cat will return to the spot and mark it again!

Playful Tips

Pet-proofing your home is a lot like baby-proofing. Like our babies, our cats and dogs are unaware of the dangers they may encounter while playing on the floor, cruising around the house and inevitably putting things in their mouths. Because what's dangerous for our pets is dangerous for our babies, as pet owners and parents it's up to us to step in and provide everyone involved with the most secure home environment. Like we've said: Making your home pet-safe creates a baby- and family-safe home as well. The two go hand in paw (sorry, we couldn't resist).

Since a pet toy is a baby toy in disguise, keep your pets and little ones safe from anything that could be picked up and swallowed—stray string, marbles, rubber bands, paper clips, coins, *you name it*—by regularly sweeping your floors. Keep your pets busy instead with "pet-specific" toys that are safe to gnaw on, tear up, and chew. See the following smart solutions for choosing the best ones.

SMART SOLUTIONS:
Making Toys Pet and Baby-Safe

- Choose trusted brands over unknown brands. You may spend a bit more but in our opinion, you're buying peace of mind that your pet is playing safe. Plus, remember that every pet toy is a potential baby toy!
- Make sure it's size-appropriate. As a general rule, avoid balls and toys smaller than your pet's jaw or that can easily break into smaller pieces that can become a choking hazard.
- Consider color. Many popular pet toys are colored with toxic dyes and decorated with lead paints. Reduce the risk of harmful exposure by generally avoiding painted toys and choosing "nontoxic" and "pet-safe" labels.
- Remove the removable risk. Buttons, plastic ears, and stretchy tails pose a choking hazard to your dog *and* your baby. Avoid toys with pieces and parts that can easily come off or fall apart when chewed and consider purchasing simple toys that are made of only one piece.
- Check the wear and tear. After a few good chewings, assess the condition of the toy. Replace toys when they start to look ragged and begin falling apart.
- Pass on the rawhides. Pets love them, but we recommend allowing your dog to have this treat only when you're around to keep a close watch. Rawhide chews should be large and thick enough that your dog cannot easily break off pieces small enough to choke on.

- Keep toys separate. Yes, they're sharing the same floor space, but it's a safe idea to keep your pet's toys out of your children's hands and mouths whenever possible. When your baby plays with a toy that your pet has had in his mouth, she runs the risk of coming into contact with bacteria and allergens that are passed through pet saliva. Make a habit of washing your child's hands with soap and water after she plays with your pet (a smart solution we've no doubt drilled into your head by now).

Low-Lying Playmates

You've created an environment that's safe for your pets, but what happens when you mix in the kids? How can all your babies play safely *together*? Making sure your pet and your baby get off to a good start takes work, but it's well worth the effort.

Q: **Dear Founding Fathers,**

I've heard about parents who, in an effort to get their pets ready for a baby, do things like play the sound of a baby crying or carry around a swaddled baby doll for their pet to see. Sorry, but this seems silly. Do tricks like this really work? Can you really prepare your pet for the arrival of a baby?

A: Dear Pregnant Pet Owner,

The answer is yes! There are lots of things (not so silly) you can do while you're preparing your pet for a new baby. OK, there's no guarantee that just because you do these things your pet will immediately love his new sibling. Building any kind of friendship takes time, but we've found that a little preparation can go a long way.

A few things we recommend: Bust out the baby gear early. Yes, it takes up space. (Get used to it!) Set up the Pack 'n Play, the bouncer, and the swing so that your pet can sniff, rub up against, and begin to get comfortable with all the new loot in the house. In other words, don't wait until you bring your baby home to rearrange the living room. If this is your first baby, consider inviting friends over who already have babies. A pet that's never been around an infant is in for a shock. The shriek of a newborn can be enough to send some pets running for cover. And finally, introduce baby smells. Because your pets have such a discerning sense of smell, it's a good idea to begin using the lotions and soaps that you will eventually use on your baby on yourself. You might also strategically place a receiving blanket or a onesie with your baby's scent on it in your pet's bed, under his food dish, or in one of his favorite hangouts. This will help your pet become familiar with the smell of your baby before she comes home—and ruins everything!

You can take all the steps in the world to prepare your pet for the arrival of your baby, but the day she comes home is often the most crucial. First impressions really do matter. Spend some time planning for that first meet and greet. Consider the smart solutions below; they can help make that first introduction between your pet and child a friendly one.

SMART SOLUTIONS:
Baby, Meet Baby!

- Single File. It's a smart idea to have Dad walk through the front door first, and greet your pet calmly and with affection. Pet and stroke him, give him a treat and reassure him that everything's cool. Once your pet is calm and secure, have Mom enter the house holding baby.
- Establish an upper hand. Have Mom sit on the couch or in a chair, holding baby close and covering his head with her hand. This communicates Mom's fierce protectiveness of the newest member of the household.
- Keep your pet on a leash and at a distance for introductions. Let your babies greet each other from across the room. If your pet doesn't act out by growling, hissing, pointing his ears back, or putting his tail down, you may slowly allow your cat or dog to wander over to baby and have a sniff.
- Avoid ground-level greetings. Never put your new baby on the ground with your pet in the same room; this may trigger your pet's defensiveness and alpha aggression. For the same reason, it's also a smart idea to keep

your dog away from your baby or toddler when they're in a walker, bouncer, or jumper—anything that brings them eye-to-eye and makes your pet appear and feel bigger than your baby.

- Send him to his room. If your dog or cat displays any negative behavior, firmly say "no." and don't hesitate to physically remove your pet from the room.

Even if the introductions go well and your pet is a perfect host, it's a smart idea to watch him for several weeks, especially when both of your babies want to share the same space. Their world has been turned upside down, so look out for odd or naughty behavior, like refusal to use the litter box, loss of appetite, excessive sleeping, and acting withdrawn. If your pet is doing any of these things, she's likely still adjusting to the new kid in town. Give your pet time to relax, and once she does, slowly begin to include her in your new daily routine. Allow your pet to follow you around the house as you do laundry, prepare bottles, and change diapers. During naps (if you're not taking one yourself), give your pet a little one-on-one attention and remind him he is still your firstborn! Over time, your pets and children will likely make great playmates, developing a lasting and loving bond. As parents we can help foster this relationship.

According to Kevin . . .

The first few months with a newborn is a loony-tunes time and your pet really feels it. Dogs feel fear, happiness, sadness, anger, possessiveness . . . even loss. I started to recognize the telltale signs of depression in Tucker not long after we brought Tyler home. He slept more than normal and played less. At one point, he even lost interest in his food. That's always a big red flag! Like a lot of pet-parents, I felt guilty—*I'd abandoned my first baby!* But one day about six months later, I found Tucker sleeping right outside the nursery. It was as if he was guarding the door! I realized then that Tucker hadn't been abandoned. He was as important to the family as ever; he'd just taken on a new role as Tyler's protective older sibling. After a while, our pets adjust.

Once your pet gets over his natural resentment for losing his spot as the center of the universe, he will become your baby's biggest protector and champion. Once I recognized this shift in the family dynamic two things happened: One, I stopped feeling so guilty, and two, I became aware of how important it was to create a safe environment for Tucker and Tyler to interact. If they were going to be BFFs, they needed the time and space to develop a lasting relationship.

By taking a common-sense approach and considering the smart solutions below, you can safely create a never-ending playdate between your children and your pets.

SMART SOLUTIONS:
Kids and Pets at Play

- Consider your pet's uniqueness. Just like people, all pets are different. Take into account your pet's training, general disposition, and mood, you can probably guess what your child's in for. Is your pet jumpy and nervous, or calm and controlled? Consider how your babies and pets will get along before planning a playdate.
- Give your pet space. Toddlers in particular love to invade our pets' space. Dog bed—mine! Kitty dish—mine! This can incite a turf war, so before your child receives an unpleasant nip, teach her about boundaries. Explain that the dog's bed, the kitty's bowl, and the pet door are off-limits.
- Avoid eye level and a leg up. Keep your dog away from your baby or toddler when they're in a walker, bouncer, or jumper—anything that brings them eye to eye, which can make some dogs defensive. Also, discourage your dog from sitting next to you on the couch or the bed if you're holding your baby. This makes dogs appear and feel bigger than your baby and may trigger alpha aggression.
- Pet gently. From early on, teach your little one to stroke your pet gently. Explain that eyes, ears, and mouths are not to be touched, and that tugging on tails and pulling on whiskers is a not-nice "no-no!"
- Play the referee. While your child is still little and learning to crawl and walk, it's not safe to leave your babies alone in the playroom. Ever. An

unintentional jab, poke, or tumble onto a foot or tail could invite a hiss, scratch, or a bite. Until your child is two years old, play the ref—stay close, keep an eye on them, and be ready to step in if needed.

- Don't force a relationship. If they just aren't into each other, that's fine. They will likely develop a relationship in time.

Q: **Dear Founding Fathers,**

My son's favorite game to play with our family dog involves messing with his dog food. He takes it out of the bowl, piece by piece, and then drops them into the water bowl—drop, plop, splash! I swear, he thinks it's the funniest thing ever. I don't see the humor and my dog doesn't either, but the bigger concern is whether playing with dog food is even safe? My guess is no. Am I right?

A: **Dear Not-so-Proud Papa,**

You're right. Your son isn't as funny as he thinks. First of all, he's crossed a line on to his dog's turf. We're surprised you haven't heard a growl or seen a couple of pinned-back ears. Dogs don't like it when anyone messes with their food! Secondly, your son may just be interested in *playing* with your dog's kibble for now, but it's only a matter of time before he pops some of it into his mouth. As with all things small, round, and hard, dog food is a potential choking hazard and that water bowl is no better—would you believe it's a drowning hazard? Also, the water dish can become a pool for nasty bacteria! And even if nothing goes directly into your son's mouth, his hands are touching a lot of dog saliva and we're guessing he's not leaving his game to wash his hands. Our advice is to put your dog's food and water in the garage, on the porch, or somewhere your son can't easily reach. Once he's a bit older, you can bring the pet food back into the house and teach him how to help care for your pets, by filling food and water bowls and offering treats. This is a fun game both your pet and child can enjoy!

Some "pet-parental" advice: To minimize icky microbial growth in your pets' dishes and bowls, change the water frequently and use a natural, plant-based, and nontoxic cleaner to routinely wash them out.

Now that you've learned a thing or two about creating a safe and healthy indoor environment for all your babies, what happens when your fur babies go outside, roll around in the dirt, and track pesticides, synthetic fertilizers, and who-knows-what-else back inside? How do you ensure the same level of safety for your babies and pets in your outdoor space without replacing your lawn with AstroTurf (and how safe is artificial grass, anyway)?

Time to take it outdoors. We'll explain how to apply everything you've learned to playing healthy, clean, and safe outside the home—in your backyard, as well as in your favorite parks and public spaces.

Smart Solutions at a Glance

Clean and Coiffed

- Significantly limit how much and how frequently your pets shed by regularly getting them into the bath.
- Choose pet shampoos and conditioners that are pH-balanced and made with plant-based ingredients like tea-tree oil, aloe, and vitamin E and omega-3 fatty acids that both moisturize fur and keep the skin and coat healthy and flake-free.
- Residual shampoo and conditioner can become an irritant, creating more shedding, more dander, more dust balls on the floor and allergens in the air.

A Buggy Situation

- Invest in a vacuum with a HEPA filter to trap animal dander and dust-mite droppings.
- Make your child's bedroom a pet-free zone while they're very young or until you can determine if your child has a pet allergy.
- Consult your vet about flea prevention and then take a minimalist approach. Pills that leave no chemical residue on your pet's coat are the safest solution.

- Pregnant women should not handle kitty litter because it increases the risk of contracting toxoplasmosis.
- Steer clear of cleaning up pet "accidents" with products containing ammonia because your pets will be drawn to the smell and mark the spot again!

Playful Tips

- Avoid painted toys and look for "nontoxic" and "pet-safe" labels.
- Replace any pet toy when it starts to fall apart or when pieces and parts can be easily chewed off.
- Keep your pet's toys out of your children's hands and mouths to reduce the risk of your child coming into contact with bacteria and allergens that are passed through saliva.
- Consider your pet's personality and temperament before allowing your babies to play together.
- Stay close, supervise their play, and be ready to step in if needed.
- Don't force a relationship. It will likely develop in time.

Step 7

A Baby-Safe World

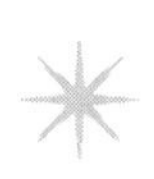

By now you're armed with plenty of tools and solutions to help you impact the health and safety of your family. You've spent the last six steps cleaning up your crib and becoming even more aware of what's going onto and into your babies and your pet's vulnerable bodies. Now we're going to show you how to clean up your outdoor spaces so that they, too, are as healthy and safe as they can be. In this step, we'll share with you what we've learned about

- Maintaining a pet- and baby-safe yard
- Growing a safe garden
- How to bug off naturally
- The healthiest way to have fun in the sun
- The secret to your baby's freedom

Green Your Outdoor Space

Remember, pound for pound, babies breathe twice as much air as we do. Their little lungs are hard at work! This puts them at a higher risk of inhaling and ingesting harmful contaminants that their developing bodies can't process and detoxify. Just as they do inside, babies and children love to crawl, play, and roll around on the ground outside the home, and this puts them in direct contact with pesticides used to control weeds, fungus, and insects in our gardens and yards. Even if you're not using them, chances are high that someone on your neighborhood is. Get this: It's estimated that homeowners apply about 78 million pounds of insecticides, herbicides, and fungicides per year to their homes, lawns, and gardens, and this doesn't include what pest control and lawn-care professionals are spraying or dusting up and down your block. And these chemicals, even in small doses, can be highly toxic to your children and pets.

How toxic are these chemicals? Pretty darn toxic. Allergic reactions linked to pesticide exposure include asthma; nausea; vomiting; diarrhea; muscle and joint pain; weakness; dizziness; ear, nose, and throat irritation; blurry vision; and mental confusion. And that's not all. Organophosphates, a class of pesticides used by exterminators and found in many household and garden products, are especially harmful to pregnant women and children. Studies show that even low-level exposure to these nasty buggers is linked to birth defects, miscarriages, and infertility, and studies indicate that pesticides can also pass from mother to child through umbilical cord blood and breast milk. The National Academy of Sciences estimates that 50 percent of lifetime pesticide exposure occurs during the *first five years of life.*

This kind of makes you rethink the importance of a weed- and pest-free yard, doesn't it? But when you think about it, this information isn't all that surprising when you consider that pesticides and herbicides are designed to *kill living things.* Why wouldn't they pose a threat to our pets and children, too?

Kevin and Keith's KEEP-OFF-THE-LAWN List

PESTICIDES

Where you'll find them: Household and garden products primarily used to control (i.e. kill) unwanted insects.

Why they're bad news: Pesticide exposure has been linked to nausea; vomiting; diarrhea; muscle and joint pain; weakness; dizziness; ear, nose, and throat irritation; blurry vision; and mental confusion. There is growing concern that exposure to organophosphates, a class of pesticides, may produce lower IQ scores in children, hyperactivity, a shortened attention span, delays in cognitive development, and difficulties with short-term memory.

HERBICIDES

Where you'll find them: Weed killer.

Why they're bad news: Herbicides are suspected to cause pregnancy problems, leading to abnormal fetal development, low birth weights, or miscarriages. They are also potential endocrine disrupters, affecting healthy growth in children.

So maybe you're thinking, "Hey, I only spray weeds and bugs in the farthest corners of my yard—completely out of harm's way. This shouldn't be a problem." While we'd like to tell you that responsible application reduces the risk of exposure, it doesn't really work that way. Pesticides and herbicides don't stay put. They easily become airborne and drift—onto your lawn where your kids and pets like to play and into your house where they can settle on your furniture and the floor. Therefore, our best parental advice is to steer clear of synthetic herbicides, pesticides, and fertilizers. Try instead the following smart solutions to safely green your outdoor space.

SMART SOLUTIONS:
A Greener Garden

- Plant native grass. When you plant grass that naturally thrives where you live, you need a whole lot less fertilizer, pesticide, water, and maintenance.
- Grow what's natural. In addition to planting native grass, consider a natural and minimal approach to landscaping.
- Pull weeds by hand. Sure, it's old school, but it's safe and effective (especially when you get your kids to lend you a hand).
- Trim your lawn. Longer blades of grass develop strong root systems, allowing them to stay greener for longer. Not only that, but longer blades also tower over, shade, and outcompete weeds. Set your mower blade two to three inches from the ground and trim just the ends.
- Clip it and leave it. When grass clippings are left on the lawn, they break down into nitrogen that feeds the soil.

Q: **Dear Founding Fathers,**

I can control what goes on in my own backyard, but what about next door? I have a sneaking suspicion that my neighbors are using pesticides and herbicides on their lawn and I'm worried about toxic "drift" and "track in." I've heard that pesticides can become airborne and attach to dust that's then tracked into every home in the neighborhood. I know it's not really my business what my neighbors do, but in this case maybe it is. It's my job to keep my children healthy and safe, but I'm not sure how to address the issue without crossing the line. What's the neighborly thing to do?

A: **Dear Want to Avoid Chemical Warfare,**

It's true that what happens on the other side of your property line can directly affect your family's health. Even on a slightly breezy day, chemicals being used on the house next door can drift into your yard or in through your windows and settle onto your surfaces and floors. Even at low levels, exposure to chemical herbicides and pesticides can have negative health effects over time. And while you don't have a lot of control over what your neighbors do or don't do, you don't have to cross the line to *draw the line.* What we mean is, there's nothing wrong with having a civilized conversation. Ask them what they're using to manage pests and treat their garden and lawn. If they're using a professional gardener or landscaper, they might not even know what products are being used on their property. Suggest they find out. Prime them with a few questions, starting with: What types of chemicals are you using? Maybe ease them into a discussion about the potential risks you know of.

If you discover that your neighbors are regularly using toxic and potentially harmful chemicals to tend their outdoor space, take the opportunity to plant a healthy seed. Offer safer alternatives. Share some of the nontoxic and effective solutions you've adopted and suggest they meet you in the middle.

In addition to learning about what's going on over your neighbor's fence, find out what's happening in the rest of the hood. Think about it: All it takes is one good rain and pesticides and herbicides run amok through the streets, easily getting on the bottoms of your shoes and in through your door. Some towns have laws that require residents to provide forty-eight-hour advance notice before using toxic chemicals on their property. Know the rules where you live. On days when chemicals may be released into the air, plan to visit friends or bring both your pets and babies indoors and close the windows. Keep them out of the yard for a good twenty-four hours after chemicals have been used. Consider pulling toys inside until the coast is clear, or at the very least hose them down before letting your little ones play with them again.

Helpful Resource: Who's Polluting?

You can get an in-depth pollution report for your county by visiting the EFD's Scorecard at www.scorecard.org. Discover if nearby power plants, factories, industrial facilities, and manufacturers are releasing chemical by-products into your community's air and water.

According to Keith . . .

In my neighborhood, if a lawn has been treated with chemicals, flags are staked on the property alerting residents that it's been recently sprayed. I've explained to my kids what these flags mean: Dangerous chemicals that can make you sick are on that lawn—keep off the grass!

My kids are outdoorsy. They both play sports and love the beach, biking, and getting dirty wherever they can. And I wouldn't want it any other way. Research shows that spending time outdoors enhances kids' motor skills, social development, attention, and activity level. It can creatively inspire them, and also chill them out. Exploring nature also helps children make sense of the world. Plus it's an inexpensive good time! For these reasons, Nicole and I encourage our kids to hit the green *a lot.* This means, however, they're at risk of being exposed to harmful chemicals and contaminants. But unless I lock them inside (which would drive us and them crazy), the most we can do when it comes to ensuring they play safe is to make them aware of any potential risks and encourage them to make smart choices and practice healthy habits—like staying off the chemically treated lawn and *washing their hands*!

I know I sound just like a (ugh!) repetitive dad, but safe outdoor play has everything to do with good hand hygiene. When my kids are playing in the backyard or in a public space, I encourage them to keep their hands out of the dirt and away from their mouths. As soon as we walk in the front door, the first thing they do is wash their hands (Nicole and I also wipe them down with an alcohol-free hand sanitizer on the ride home). Washing hands sounds so simple (because it is), but it's a smart solution that makes a *huge* difference in limiting their exposure to toxic elements outside the home.

Walk this way

When it comes to avoiding toxic outdoor insecticides and herbicides, it's not just a matter of what our children's hands can get into. As parents, we also have to be aware of what our small human and animal residents track indoors on the bottoms of their feet and paws. The truth is that most of the dust and dirt in your house has traveled inside on the bottom of someone's feet. Even the most consciously minded track in dirt, and trust us—those fine particles collect *everywhere.* And the thing about dirt is it's magnetic. You've heard of the Law of Attraction, right? Dirt attracts more dirt.

Even if you sweep and vacuum often (a smart solution we applaud), dirt particles have a way of collecting and multiplying like bunnies in your house every time you walk through the door. And if the dirt coming in on your shoes, your baby's feet, or your pet's paws has toxic residue, guess what? It's getting everywhere in the house, too.

We don't mean to freak you out, but since we're going there . . . A study conducted at the University of Arizona found that most people's shoes carry about nine different species of bacteria on them at any given moment. If that's not gross enough, shoes are a bacterial petri dish—bacteria actually live longer on our shoes than in most other places, and are continuously being replenished as we walk around outside, through buildings, and in public restrooms. Yuck! When *Good Morning America* looked into it in 2008, they found far more bacteria on shoes (literally tens of millions per shoe) than on a public toilet seat. Yeah. You get the idea. Our feet are dirty, so get into a regular (as in every day!) habit of taking off your shoes as soon as you walk through the door. Wipe them down and leave them in a basket, or better yet, on the front porch.

Q: Dear Founding Fathers,

I've heard that some porches, decks, lawn furniture, and play sets can be unsafe for my children to play on. Should I be worried about my outdoor space? I thought wood was safe.

A: Dear Wood Worrier,

Decks, lawn, porch, and patio furniture are sometimes made of pressure-treated wood that is treated with chemicals to ward off wood-chomping bugs and prevent rot. One of the more popular chemical combos used in pressure-treated wood is chromated copper arsenate (CCA), which contains arsenic, a known human carcinogen. So the legitimate worry is that decks, porches, outdoor play sets, and furniture treated with CCA can leach chemicals out of the wood and onto your children's hands.

Before you declare all hands off deck, know that if your deck was built in the last ten years, your family is likely free from harm. In 2003, the EPA banned the use of CCA in pressure-treated wood in outdoor furniture, picnic tables at parks, and wood chips in playgrounds. A water-based wood preservative called alkaline copper quaternary (ACQ) took its place and so far it's proving to be safe.

On the other hand, if your deck's more than a decade old, or if you're not sure about your child's wooden play set and you'd like to play it baby-safe, apply two liberal coats of an oil-based sealant to the pieces in question, and be sure your kids wash their hands after eating off or playing on anything suspicious. Reapplication is a must to keep CCA contained, so slap on a fresh coat at least once a year. If that's more maintenance than you want to deal with and you'd rather start from the ground up, consider buying pieces made out of natural untreated wood. Cedar, redwood, and teak are great choices.

Q: Dear Founding Fathers,

We built a play structure for my kids that I know is safe. It's made out of wood that's been treated with a nontoxic water-based solution and my husband screwed and bolted every piece into place by hand. We spent a good deal of money and time building this backyard playground for our kids, but they prefer the public playground down the street. It's much bigger, has fancy features like a climbing wall and tunnel slides, and many of the neighborhood kids play there. I don't want to be a total stick-in-the-mud and the only mom on the block who fences my kids in, but I've heard too many scary stories about toxins in public play structures (which is why we built our own!). But I'm losing the battle—my kids are on strike. They're refusing to play in our backyard. Before I accept defeat and turn my kids loose, how can I know if it's safe?

A: Dear Losing Ground,

You can still win this backyard battle. Make a deal with your kids that if you determine that the playground down the street is 100 percent safe, you'll let them play there. Once they agree to your conditions (and they will; your house, your rules), take a trip down to the park and have a look around. Check for signs of rust and chipping paint. This is a lead alert! Also consider the surface area around the playground. Trips, spills, and falls are inevitable (we're talking kids here), and concrete and asphalt are far less forgiving than wood chips, rubber, gravel, or sand.

Did you know that U.S. hospitals treat as many as 500,000 children every year for playground-related injuries, of which more than half are falls onto hard surfaces? *Where's the fun in that?* The good news is that whether they're in the backyard or down the street, your kids are likely playing safe. Most of the newer play structures are built with recycled materials like steel, plastic, and sustainable wood, and treated with nontoxic sealants and paints.

Dig In

Enough of the backyard horrors! Outdoor time should be fun, right? So, let's talk about one of our favorite activities to do outdoors that's not only healthy and safe, but makes children happy—gardening.

According to Keith . . .

My family loves to eat local, organic, fresh produce, and we're also passionate about growing the food we eat. My wife and I started a backyard garden when Zach was four years old. It began as a weekend hobby that we thought would be fun for the kids and also teach them something valuable—how our food starts from a seed and grows into a plant that we eventually harvest, cook, and bring to our dinner table. The whole farm-to-table thing.

By the end of first season, I'd gotten really into it and decided to take it to another level by becoming a USDA-certified organic grower so I'd know exactly how to grow fruits and vegetables without toxic chemicals (and yield bigger and more fruitful crops. Yeah. I'm competitive!). Gardening has become a huge part of our family life and over the years, we've produced hundreds of tomatoes, cucumbers, beets, green beans, and strawberries. Last year, we grew artichokes, broccoli, and cauliflower. This year, we're going for zucchini and red, green, and yellow peppers. The kids get a kick out of seeing the literal fruits of their labor. I often find them after school showing their friends how to pick a green bean or pull up a carrot. They'll bring their fresh produce inside to eat for their afternoon snack. Really—how cool is that?

Planting a garden creates an awesome opportunity to connect with your food, have fun with your kids, and "green" your outdoor space. Here are a few planting ideas and smart solutions to consider before digging in.

SMART SOLUTIONS:

Growing a Garden

- Know what you're planting on. What's the condition of your soil? Try to find out if any toxic chemicals were used in your outdoor space before you moved in. Municipal or town records, and sometimes the local historical society, can usually shed some light. If you're concerned that your soil may be tainted, consider planting your garden aboveground in planter boxes. This smart precautionary move creates a definitive barrier between the food you're growing and the existing soil.

- Avoid engineered, pressure-treated wood. When building borders and garden beds, stick with natural wood that hasn't been treated with chemicals that can leach into the soil and get onto your or your little ones' hands or contaminate your plants.
- Keep your friends and veggies close. Even if your yard is chemical-free, it doesn't mean the lawn next door is. If your neighbor is using pesticides along your shared fence, they may be passing over into your yard. Plant your garden at a significant distance away from the property line, and suggest your neighbors try a few nontoxic alternatives (it doesn't hurt to ask!).
- Garden by hand. Keep weeds safely under control by pulling them up by hand and lining garden beds with newspaper or cardboard. Weed-blocking fabrics work well, too. Top your garden beds with organic mulch to suppress weeds (without light they can't grow!). Mulch also helps your plants retain water.
- Bug off naturally. Crushed eggshells scattered around the perimeter of your garden are your best defense against slugs; they won't cross the line. Erecting a trestle for vine-growing plants will maximize space and keep fruits and veggies off the ground and away from unwanted pests. Finally, bug off naturally by inviting ladybugs into your garden (they love to eat aphids) and adding colorful flowers like marigolds and zinnias, which attract predator insects that eat the bugs with an appetite for your plants.

Bug Off Naturally!

Now that you know how to naturally attack the pests that like to make a meal of your tomatoes, what about the bugs that like to invade our personal space? Mosquitoes and gnats—shoo! Flies, roaches, and ants—stop bugging me! As tempting as it may be to declare war (especially when hosting a backyard barbecue), it's not a great idea to snuff them out chemically. Not only do pesticides mess with the environment (some bugs develop a resistance, making for a much bigger pest problem and an out-of-whack ecosystem), but they are also a big-time menace to us—they're highly toxic to our children and pets.

Take deet, for example, a chemical commonly found in bug repellents. Deet is very effective at getting the job done. It kills bugs, but if inhaled by an adult, deet can cause eye irritation, skin rash, hives, redness, and swelling. If swallowed, it can attack the central nervous system and cause disorientation, nausea—even seizures. Imagine the effect it could have on your babies. No thanks! The American Academy of Pediatrics assures us that small amounts of deet applied in the "right" way can be safe, but we'd rather be extra safe than right.

The truth is, you don't need a poisonous weapon to repel bugs. If you are tempted to spray your child with something as powerful as deet, we urge you to think about the real risks. If we're talking about areas with high rates of Lyme disease and West Nile virus, that's one thing, but most day-to-day outdoor settings aren't this risky. So except for extreme circumstances like traveling to a country where malaria or dengue fever is a real concern, nontoxic products made with essential aromatic oils like citronella, peppermint, rosemary leaf, lemongrass, soybean, and geranium are not only repellent to insects, especially mosquitoes, but in the right combination are gentle on your baby's skin. Plus, believe it or not, they can rival the efficacy of most chemical solutions. In other words, with a natural repellent you can bug-off safely and enjoy spending time outdoors with your family without worrying about getting munched.

We believe the best defense against bugs isn't full-blown extermination, but safely *controlling* them. So in addition to throwing out insect repellents with harsh chemicals like deet (really, if it's on the list of ingredients, it's got to go), and choosing a nontoxic alternative, consider the following smart solutions.

SMART SOLUTIONS:
Shoo Bug!

- Eliminate standing water. Pools of water are breeding grounds for mosquitoes. Take a walk around your outdoor space and dump out any water collecting in buckets, toys, pots, or gutters. Inside, wipe up spills under the fridge, be careful not to overwater houseplants, and make sure you fix leaky pipes. Standing water inside the home attracts roaches and other critters.
- Blow them away. Mosquitoes and gnats can't fly against a current, so turn up the outdoor fan and enjoy the bug-free breeze.
- Cover up. Slip your little ones into long-sleeved pants and shirts and

spray their clothes with repellent. Consider loose and thin clothing that easily breathes, especially when it's 90° F, or expect a meltdown! Cover up with light-colored solid fabrics (many insects are attracted to dark colors and loud prints). Tuck your child's pants into his socks and dress him in closed-toe shoes to prevent tick bites.

- Ditch the sweet smells. Another reason to wash your babies with fragrance-free soaps and shampoos is that they will attract fewer pests. A child that smells like a sweet, fruity treat is good enough to eat!
- Keep food sealed. Pests are attracted to food and garbage (one man's trash is another bug's treasure), so once the picnic is over, throw food far away from where your children are playing and seal up any leftovers.
- Stay indoors at dawn and dusk. When the light's just right, mosquitoes are out in force and hungry, so don't schedule outdoor playtime during mosquitoes' mealtime!

Bouncing back from a bite

You can take every precaution, but from time to time bug bites just happen. They're an unavoidable rite of passage. Do you remember your first sting? We do, and it wasn't sweet! The first step to treating an insect sting is removing the stinger from the skin if you can find it. Once the stinger is removed, wash the infected area thoroughly with soap and water. Relieve any swelling by pressing an ice pack or cold compress to the site. Do your best to keep your child from scratching (good luck with that), because this can worsen the swelling and break the skin, allowing for infection-causing bacteria to enter the body. If you notice anything suspicious develop—like more redness, swelling, or pain, and especially a fever—call your pediatrician ASAP.

While it's no fun when bugs bite, in most cases an insect sting will swell or a bug bite will itch for a day or two and then it'll be over—the bump will disappear and your child will be off playing again.

Q: **Dear Founding Fathers,**

I'm less concerned with the bugs outside than the ones inside our home. I feel like I'm doing everything right—I keep our floors clear of crumbs that could attract roaches and other bugs. Our garbage pail has a tight-fitting lid on it and we take it out religiously. We also keep our food stored and sealed in either plastic or glass containers, put the dog food up overnight and *still,* roaches, ants, and spiders show up at my door. I'm starting to lose it! How can we naturally and safely control bugs inside the home?

A: **Dear Bugging Out,**

You're clearly not a food pantry, but the bugs are lining up for a handout anyway. They might finally get the hint and go elsewhere if you cut them off at the entrance. Try caulking any cracks or holes around your baseboards and cabinets. You might also try neem oil, which has been used for centuries in organic farming practices, as well as by cultures worldwide as an organic pesticide. It can be sprayed in and around the home, near doors, or along baseboards and works as a repellent. Garlic oil can be used in much the same way.

If these tricks don't work, and you feel like you need to take stronger action, consider putting a few bait houses around or injecting an insecticidal gel into cracks where bugs might be making their entrance. Be aware that the chemicals in both a gel and a bait house can be toxic and should be kept far out of reach of your children and pets (under the stove, fridge, or behind the couch are good places to set up house). Because they're contained, these chemicals are less likely to become airborne, which puts them on the low end of the risk scale. Still, use sparingly.

Helpful Resource: Integrated Pest Management

Employ services that use Integrated Pest Management (IPM). Their philosophy is that pests should be controlled, not eliminated, using the least toxic products and substances in the smallest possible quantities.

Fun in the Sun

If your child is playing outdoors, then there's no way around it—she's being exposed to the sun and, as we talked about earlier in Step 3, its rays (even on overcast days) are extra dangerous to our little ones, especially to sensitive infant skin, which burns fast and has a tough time recovering from a burn. Whatever their age, if your child is spending any amount of time at the park, pool, or on the front porch, then sunscreen is a must. According to current estimates, one in five people will develop skin cancer in their lifetime. It's the most common form of cancer in the United States, with more than 3.5 million cases diagnosed every year, and rates are increasing. Furthermore, sun damage at an early age creates a higher risk of melanoma, the deadliest type of skin cancer, later in life. Yup, that's the sizzling truth.

With so many options available, it can be difficult to know which sunscreen to use to protect your baby. Which ones are safe and gentle? Which are the most effective? How much protection does your baby really need? When choosing suncare products, we recommend carefully selecting a broad-spectrum sunscreen that is mineral-based, nontoxic, and fragrance-free. Here's why: Chemical sunscreens work by absorbing and deactivating the sun's rays, preventing them from harming your skin, but many contain toxic ingredients (like parabens, sulfates, and phthalates, to name just a few) that are simply too harsh for your baby's skin. Take oxybenzone, for example, a chemical that can be found in many adult and baby sunscreens. While effective at absorbing the sun's rays, oxybenzone is also absorbed directly into your baby's skin and bloodstream and has raised more than a few concerned eyebrows about its potential hormone-altering and carcinogenic side effects. To best protect your baby's sensitive skin, we recommend choosing a mineral-based sunscreen that works by reflecting and scattering the sun's rays, rather than absorbing them. Titanium dioxide and zinc oxide turn you into a human reflector, bouncing light off your body. *Kapow!*

Q: Dear Founding Fathers,

I'm confused. I thought mineral oil was basically liquid petroleum. I assumed it was bad because it blocks the body's natural ability to breathe, sweat, and release toxins. Could you clarify?

A: Dear Minerally Muddled,

Hey, good catch! To help clear up any confusion, "mineral oil" and "mineral-based" are two very different things. You are correct that mineral oil coats and clogs the skin, and is not a great skincare ingredient especially for babies' thin and sensitive skin. Not only does it block the skin's ability to breathe, but mineral oil can also produce a nasty sunburn! "Mineral-based" is very different. Natural minerals like zinc oxide and titanium dioxide reflect the sun's harmful rays really well. We love mineral-based sunscreens because they are not only effective and safe, but they also generally last longer than chemical sunscreens. Because they don't need to be absorbed into the skin, they can be applied to your child's face and hands right before heading out the door, and just like that—your baby's covered!

Kevin and Keith's

NOT-SO-FUN-IN-THE-SUN List

PARA-AMINOBENZOIC ACID (PABA)

Where you'll find it: A once-common sunscreen ingredient.

Why it's bad news: Research indicates PABA has carcinogenic potential. PABA derivatives are now more commonly used, but these too may cause side effects, including allergic dermatitis. There are also concerns that they may cause biochemical or cellular-level changes in people who use them regularly.

OXYBENZONE

Where you'll find it: In many sunscreens.

Why it's bad news: Oxybenzone is an active chemical ingredient that is absorbed through the skin and into the bloodstream. It contaminates the bodies of 97 percent of Americans, according to research by the Centers for Disease Control and Prevention. It's a suspected hormone disrupter.

The sun-protection factor

By choosing a "broad-spectrum" sunscreen, you and your children are protected from both UVB and UVA. What's the difference? UVB causes sunburn. UVA penetrates more deeply, causing aging and wrinkles. Both increase your risk of skin cancer. As for SPF, the American Cancer Society and most dermatologists recommend SPF 15 for general, but limited, sun exposure, and SPF 30 if you spend any time outdoors, especially between the hours of 10:00 A.M. and 4:00 P.M. when the sun is most intense. We agree that in most cases, a sunscreen with an SPF 30 is healthy, safe, and provides the right balance of protection, and yet, given that our infants' and children's skin is so thin and sensitive, we say—go higher, baby! In our opinion, a broad-spectrum sunscreen with SPF 50 provides excellent protection for your little ones—98 percent of the sun's rays are either reflected or absorbed. That's significant coverage!

Q: **Dear Founding Fathers,**

Why stop at SPF 50 when there are sunscreens on the market for our children with SPF 100+? Doesn't the higher number mean it provides more protection against the sun?

A: **Dear Confused by the Numbers,**

You'd think a sunscreen with an SPF of 100+ would be twice as powerful and give you twice the protection as a sunscreen with an SPF of 50+. But this isn't the case. The reality is that once you reach SPF 50, the gain in protection is so incremental it's negligible. Properly applied, SPF 50 sunscreen blocks 98 percent of harmful rays and SPF 100 blocks 99 percent. We're talking *fractions of a percentage.* Plus, would you believe that sunscreens that boast high SPFs can actually be irritating to the skin? That's because for manufacturers to make such high and bold SPF claims, more chemicals must be added to the formula. As far as we're concerned, and most dermatologists will agree, higher SPF sunscreens are more about marketing and money, not protection. Also they often give parents a false sense of security ("We put on 100 SPF sunscreen! We're 100 percent covered! We can stay out in the sun longer!"), when really, your best protection is to reapply a lower SPF-rated sunscreen (no lower than 15 and no higher than 50) every two hours as part of your daily routine.

Maximize your coverage. Get in the habit of taking a tube of sunscreen everywhere you go and consider applying these smart solutions before heading out for a day in the sun.

SMART SOLUTIONS:

Fun in the Sun

- Apply generously. Before leaving the house, apply sunscreen generously, especially to sensitive areas—nose, ears, hands, neck, and shoulders. Reapply every two hours, at least. Sunscreen breaks down over time and is easily washed off. If your little fish likes a plunge in the pool, use common sense and reapply more often than that. No sunscreen is truly waterproof. Some are water "resistant," but they still eventually wash off. Look for products with forty to eighty minutes of water resistance, and when their time is up, blow your whistle and reapply.

- Avoid a sunscreen containing bug repellent. Many bug repellents contain deet, a harsh chemical that can be absorbed into the skin and cause neurotoxic effects. Deet is bad news and not safe to smear on your baby's skin. Also, sunscreens need to be reapplied every couple of hours, whereas insect repellents, even those that are deet-free, should not be applied with such regularity.
- Wear a hat. Cover your little one's head and ears with a hat, and dress her in protective clothing with built-in sun filters (look for labels that say UPF 40–50+). Loose and thin long-sleeved shirts and pants also work well to block the sun, and can reduce the likelihood of heat rash, that irritating, pimply skin eruption that often shows up in the sensitive folds and creases of the skin, on the tummy, and the backside. Also, consider a pair of shades with 99 percent UVA/UVB protection.
- Between 10:00 A.M. and 4:00 P.M. stay indoors. These are the hottest hours of the day, so stay out of the sun as much as possible during this peak time. Or at least under an umbrella.
- Stick to the shade. Keep babies under six months old out of direct sunlight. Park them under a shady tree. Sun umbrellas and stroller canopies are both great investments.

- Ignore the weather. Just because it's overcast doesn't mean the sun isn't hard at work on your skin. Cloudy, rainy, foggy, or sunny—every day is a sunscreen day!
- Pucker up. While we agree your baby's lips are adorably perfect, it turns out they're also super delicate and need your help. Lips are often neglected when it comes to sunscreen, but they have as few as ten layers of skin, compared with twenty or more elsewhere on your body. The American Academy of Dermatology suggests wearing an SPF 15+ lip balm for the best protection.
- Set an example. Wear sunscreen yourself and your child will come to understand that protecting yourself from the sun is just something we do to be healthy, happy, and safe.

According to Keith . . .

I coach my son's soccer team, and when we're playing tournaments, I become a tyrant about sunscreen. The boys know I won't even let them on the field unless they're properly covered. At every game, I have a stash of sunscreen at the ready to hand out to anyone who isn't protected. Toward the end of last season, the guys started giving me a hard time, calling themselves *Team Sunscreen*. Hey, whatever it takes. Team sports aren't only about building strength and discipline; they're also an opportunity to pass on safe solutions that kids can take off the field. Listen to the coach!

In the event that your child does get a burn (the sun has a way of getting through!), apply a cool compress to the tender area or draw a cool bath for your little one to soak in. Push plenty of fluids and stick to the shade or stay indoors for a few days. Pure aloe vera, mango butter, and calendula are known for their healing properties, so you may consider dabbing a little onto your child's hot spots. Just be cautious of allergic sensitivity before smearing it all over.

You can't have fun in the sun without reliable sunscreen, and that goes for parents, too. Moms take note: Applying a sunscreen with an SPF 15, which filters 92 percent of the sun's UV light, is the equivalent of applying seven layers of foundation and fourteen dustings of face powder. Save yourself some face time by skipping the makeup (you're beautiful without it!) and apply an SPF 15 sunscreen instead.

Splash safely

Sunscreen and pool safety go hand in hand. Long hours in the sun, minimal clothing, reflection from the water—it goes without saying that your baby's health and safety depend on applying and reapplying sunscreen. From head to toe, from toe to head! But that's not all. Once your baby's covered, before she dive-bombs into the pool, take a moment to consider one more thing: chlorine. Nearly every pool is filled with it. Chlorine, along with other chemicals, is added to water to kill bacteria, which is a good thing. Pools are swimming with sweat, dirt, sunscreen, cosmetics (and other unmentionables) that get into the water. Reducing your children's risk of exposure to bacteria is smart, but extended exposure to chlorine, whether it's inhaled or absorbed into the skin, can be irritating to sensitive skin, eyes, and lungs. You know those red eyes you get after a long day at the pool? That's chlorine at work! Is it deadly? No. Should your child be submerged in it every day of her summer vacation? Probably not. If you ask us—the pool is too much fun to give up on hot days, so use your best judgment. As a general safe solution, after a day of poolside play, throw your babies in the bathtub as soon as you can (they're already waterlogged, what's one more plunge?). Scrub your little one until the residual chlorine and chemical by-products are washed down the drain.

According to Kevin . . .

I live on the East Coast where summers are hot. How unpopular would I be if I banned my kids from pools? Not to mention, we have one in our backyard. But since learning how chlorine can irritate the skin and be harmful to our children's lungs, Ali and I decided a couple of years ago to convert our backyard pool to a saltwater pool. It's safer than a chlorinated pool, which means more swim time. So yeah, our house is pretty popular in the summer.

That said, a pool may be cool, but it's a big-time responsibility. A child can slip underwater in seconds, and lose consciousness and sustain permanent brain damage in less than four minutes. It happens that fast! After learning this statistic, Ali and I made a pact when the boys were little to never leave our kids unattended at the pool, whether it was the shallow end of a regular-sized swimming pool or a small kiddie pool with just a few inches of water. Even if the boys were wearing their water wings or swim vests, we made it a habit to never turn our backs. It can be easy to slip into a false sense of security when you're at a pool with a trained lifeguard or with other responsible parents on "pool duty," but the difference between safe and scary is seconds, so we never take the risk.

Safety = Freedom!

As parents, it's our job to be there to keep our babies safe. Not just so they are protected, but so that they are free to satisfy their curiosity and play and explore their world safely. But as they get older, we just can't be there *all the time.* We start dropping them off at day care and then school, sending them to summer camp—and one day we realize that they'd rather play with their friends down the street than with us, and our children are more or less out of our hands. At that point, we have to take a deep breath, put on our brave Mommy and Daddy faces, and trust other caregivers and adults to help keep them out of harm's way. But more than that, we have to trust that our children can make smart choices on their own.

After spending so much of your valuable time and energy making your home, car, backyard, and every conceivable place your child may touch out in the world baby-safe, it might feel uncomfortable, even scary, to consider taking a step back from safeguarding your child's life and handing some of the responsibility over to them. Have little fear. You've already taken the most important steps you can to ensure that your children will make choices that are healthy, clean, and safe when they're outside your reach—by becoming an *example* of healthy, clean, and safe yourself. Remember, monkey see, monkey do—so when you embrace a lifestyle that's healthy, apply smart solutions that are clean and safe, chances are very, very good that your children will do as you do—even when you aren't there to proudly see it for yourself.

According to Kevin and Keith . . .

We're often on the road, but we never stop being dads. At our age, travel can take its toll on the body, especially on healthy eating. To combat the extra weight we're both prone to putting on (the cookie-eating contests don't help) we started running together in every city we visit. Not only does this help keep us fit, but it gives us an opportunity to connect with and enjoy the places we visit on a neighborhood-by-neighborhood level. We particularly love running in Minneapolis, Austin, San Diego, and Louisville. Over the years, our on-the-road running partnership became such an enjoyable habit, we decided to bring it back home. When we're not traveling, we run together on Long Island, often with our kids in tow. There are five little ones now, including a newborn who likes the view from the jogging stroller. Baby Ashton sees all the sights without breaking a sweat. It's a pretty sweet life! On particularly hot days or if we've been hitting the pavement for a while, one of the older kids will inevitably slow down and remind us of how much she liked to be pushed when she was younger (another way of saying, "Dad, can we wrap this up?"). Because we both believe in finishing what we started, one of us will inevitably say, "Yes, but now you're big and strong and running alongside us. Isn't that awesome?" We know how we may provoke our kids when we drop little wisdom bombs like this, but an eye roll is OK by us as long as we get the results we want. When we're nearing the end of our run, we hope our fatherly speeches will give them that extra push they need to cross the finish line. As they've gotten older, we see our kids make smart, independent choices that allow them the freedom to play hard, grow, and thrive out in the world without taking a fall (or, when they do, recover quickly and confidently). That's the whole point of being baby-safe from the start, right?

Step 7: A Baby-Safe World

Smart Solutions at a Glance

Green Your Outdoor Space

- Steer clear of synthetic herbicides, pesticides, and fertilizers.
- Plant native grass and consider a natural and minimal approach to landscaping.
- On days when chemicals may be released into the air, plan to visit friends or bring both your pets and babies indoors and close the win-

dows. Keep them out of the yard for a good twenty-four hours and be sure to hose down their outdoor toys before they play with them again.

- Make a habit of taking off your shoes as soon as you walk through the door.

Dig In

- If you're concerned that your soil may be tainted with pesticides or herbicides, consider planting your garden aboveground in planter boxes.
- When building borders and garden beds, stick with natural wood that hasn't been treated with chemicals.
- If your neighbor is using pesticides along your shared fence, plant your garden at a significant distance away from the property line, and suggest your neighbors try a few nontoxic alternatives.

Bug Off Naturally!

- Crushed eggshells scattered around the perimeter of your garden are your best defense against slugs. Plant flowers like marigolds and zinnias, which attract predator insects that eat the bugs with an appetite for your plants.
- Nontoxic repellents made with essential aromatic oils like citronella, peppermint, rosemary leaf, lemongrass, soybean, and geranium in the right combination are gentle on your baby's skin.
- Eliminate standing water both inside and outside your home.
- Slip your little ones into long-sleeved shirts and pants and spray their clothes with repellent. Consider staying indoors at dawn and dusk.

Fun in the Sun

- Choose a nonchemical, broad-spectrum sunscreen that is mineral-based and fragrance-free.
- A broad-spectrum sunscreen with SPF 50 provides the most protection for your little ones—98 percent of the sun's rays are either reflected or absorbed.
- Before leaving the house, apply sunscreen generously and reapply every two hours, at least. Between 10 A.M. and 4 P.M. stay indoors or stick to the shade.

Safety = Freedom!

- When you embrace a lifestyle that's healthy, clean, and safe, chances are very good that your children will do as you do—even when you aren't there to proudly see it for yourself.

Acknowledgments

In the early days, building the babyganics business, we did everything ourselves—from coming up with product concepts to designing packaging and labels, from making cold sales calls to answering phones. But as the business grew, we learned we couldn't do it alone. Babyganics was our baby, but it took a lot of people to finally deliver her into the world. The same is true for this book. We might be the proud dads, but this book had a lot of "midwives" critical to the delivery.

First, we need to thank our *amazing* agent (Wow! We have a literary agent!?),

Yfat Reiss Gendell, at Foundry Literary + Media who believed we had a book in us and shepherded the idea from conception to delivery. Also, a big thanks to the whole Foundry team, including editorial assistant Erica Walker, foreign rights director Kirsten Neuhaus, and Sara DeNobrega.

As any one of our former English teachers will tell you, we're not exactly Hemingway and Fitzgerald. Fortunately, our co-author, Samantha Rose, stayed wide awake during her English classes! She spent hours with us, listening to what's in our heads and our hearts, and turned our words and advice into this essential go-to guide for parents. Thanks also to Julie Cucchi for always keeping the babyganics brand on the brain, and for helping Samantha capture our voice and translate it onto the page.

Thanks to all the people at Ballantine including our editor Marnie Cochran, her able assistant Nina Shield, publisher Libby McGuire, associate publisher Richard Callison, production editor Jennifer Rodriguez, editorial director Jennie Tung, and Maggie Oberrender and Susan Corcoran, for their relentless marketing and publicity, and to the Ballantine sales team for believing in and selling this book.

We couldn't have spent the time and effort necessary to create this book without the invaluable support, dedication, and hard work of our babyganics family. Everyone who works with us day in and day out does such an amazing job at running the business; it allows us to tackle projects like this. Lindsay Joyce gets a special shout-out for being the ringmaster of the whole circus of people who needed to be corralled, cajoled, and prodded into adding contributions to the thinking, writing, and research of this book.

Thanks also to our dedicated team of technical experts and advisors who help us develop our products and give us the deeper knowledge we need to advise parents as they make their homes baby-safe. Special thanks to our director of product development, Robin Forbes; our director of Research and Development, Ash Gandhi; and our medical director, Dr. Morris Nejat, for their wisdom, dedication, and patience. Thanks to our mentors, advisors, and godfathers who have believed in us since our brand was just a baby itself: Marty Fogelman, Donald Lorberbaum, Dick Wenz, Paul Desiderioscioli, and Ken Brous. And finally, thanks to all the mothers and fathers who work joyfully and tirelessly (even when they're ridiculously tired!) and who join us in our mission to make this a safe and healthy world where babies are free to explore, discover, grow, and thrive.

Index

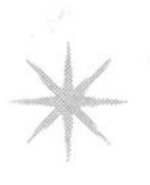

A
Advantage, 215–16
Agency for Toxic Substances and Disease Registry, 22
air-conditioning systems, 17–18
air fresheners, 19–22
air quality
  county reports, 237
  indoor, 14–22, 42–43, 45, 55–56, 80, 213–14
  time-of-day variation in, 16
alcohol-based products, 68, 76, 101
alkaline copper quaternary, 240
allergies
  food, 174–75
  pets and, 207, 213–14
  reaction to pesticides, 232–33
  see also eczema
American Academy of Pediatrics, 49, 156–57, 200
American Association of Poison Control Centers, 71, 76

American Dental Association, 200
American Grassfed Association, 171
ammonia, 65–66, 212, 218
Anna Sova paint, 42
anti-aging products, 8
antibacterial and antimicrobial products, 64–66, 68, 74–79, 100–101, 180
Apple Park toys, 141
apples, 31
arsenic, 240
Art & Creative Material Institute, 135
artificial coloring, 170
artificial sweeteners, 172
art supplies, 135
asparagus, 31
aspartame, 172
asthma, 15
avocados, 31

B

B. Toys, 141
baby bottles, 28, 72–74
babyganics, xii–xiv, 73, 106–7, 113–14, 120
baby gear
  baby-safe approach to purchasing, 146–47, 161
  product reviews, 146
  see also car seats; high chairs; strollers
baby oil, 109–10
baby powder, 124–25
baby-safe environment
  challenge of creating, xvi–xvii
  evaluating products for, xvii–xx
  goals of, xi–xii
  seven steps to, xv–xvi
bacteria and germs
  antibacterial and antimicrobial products for, 64–66, 68, 74–79, 100–101
  in baby wipe warmers, 126
  basic baby-safe practices for avoiding, 126–27
  in carpeting, 44
  on dishcloths and sponges, 74
  in food, 38–40
  food prep to avoid, 187–89
  homemade cleaning products to destroy, 84–85
  in humidifiers, 105
  in pools, 258
  practices for avoiding baby's exposure to, 95–96, 97–101
  on shoes, 239
  on toys and playthings, 142–46
  use of chlorine bleach against, 64–65
  see also infections and communicable diseases
baking soda, 21–22, 85, 125
balls, 139
Bambu, 192
BareEscentuals, 10
bathing
  basic baby-safe practices in, 127
  bathwater swallowed by baby during, 114–15
  cleaning toys after, 143–44
  foaming and sudsy products for, 111–14
  learning to drink from a cup during, 115
  for pets, 207–10, 228
  tub cleaning products, 82–84
bathroom, cleaning, 66–67, 82–84, 89–90
batteries, 137–38
bedding materials, 46–50, 214
bee stings, 247–48

beeswax, 110
Belli, 10
Benjamin Moore Pristine Eco Spec Paint, 42
Bisphenol A, 132, 135, 190–91
  health risks from, 28
  in plastic water bottles, 27–28
  potential sources of, 28
Blabla, 141
bleach, xix–xx, 64–65
  in diapers, 121
blocks, building, 139
Bobble products, 28
body lotion and washes, 7, 8, 67–68, 112–13
books, children's, 140
bovine growth hormone, 178–79
BPA, 132, 135, 190. *See also Bisphenol A*
breast milk
  benefits of, 179–80
  risk of contaminants in, 38, 179–80
bubble bath, 7, 67–68, 111–14
bug repellent strategies, 245–47
bumGenius, 117
bumper pads, 49–50
butterfish, 34

C

cabbage, 31
calamari, 34
calcium, 178, 179
candles, 19–20, 21
canned goods, 28
cantaloupe, 31
carbon monoxide detectors, 17
carpeting, 8, 44–45
car seats, 131, 149–53
castille soap, 85
catfish, 34
cats, 209–10, 216–17
caustic soda, 66–67
celery, 31
Centers for Disease Control, 200
changing table, 50–52
chapped skin, 110
char, 34
Charlie Banana, 117
cheese, 39
chemical safety testing, 61
Child Trek, 142
chloramine gas, 65–66
chlorine, 64–65, 114, 257–58
choking hazards, 136–37, 219
chromated copper arsenate, 240
clams, 34
cleaning products, home
  for carpets and rugs, 45
  labeling of, 68–70
  preparing home for baby's arrival, 59–60
  products to avoid, 60–72
  see also soaps and cleansers
cling wraps, 191, 192
clothing
  to avoid skin irritation, 105–6
  for protection from insects, 246–47
  for sun protection, 111, 255
cod, 34
Comfortis, 215–16
computer electronics, 155–59, 161
Consumer Product Safety Commission, 50, 130

cooking
  avoiding germs in, 38–40, 99
  cleaning work area for, 40, 187–88
  cutting boards, 188–89
  microwave, 191–92
  pots and pans, 189–90, 202
  preparing produce for, 33
  teaching children about, 192–93
  see also food and diet
corn, 32
cornstarch, 125
cosmetics and skincare products
  for babies, 101–3, 106–10
  good choices for, 10–14, 55
  for pets, 206–7
  potential toxins in, 6–9, 67–68, 102, 108–10
  during pregnancy, 5–14
  sunscreens and sunblocks, 110–11
CPR training, 71
crab, 35
crawfish, 35
cribs and bassinets, 46–50, 54
Crocodile Creek, 142
croup, 16–17
cucumbers, 31
cutting boards, 188–89

D

dairy products, 39, 178–80
day care
  evaluating facilities for, 98
  exposure to germs and infections in, 98
  good hygiene practices in, 98–100
DEA, 112–13
deet, 245, 255
dental care, 200–201
deodorants, 6, 7, 8, 66, 68
Department of Agriculture, 12
Department of Energy, 87
Department of Health and Human Services, 22, 170
diapers
  average baby's use of, 118
  baby's sensitivity to, 91–92
  basic baby-safe practices for, 128
  changing, 125–26
  cloth, 116–17, 128
  disposable, 117–21, 128
  expense of, 116
  flushable, 117
  hygienic practices for handling, 99
  overnight, 121–22
  potential toxins in, 7
  rash from use of, 122–25
  superabsorbent, 122
diethanolamine, 112–13
dioxane, 109, 112
dioxins, 181
dishcloths and scrubbers, 74
dish soap, 67–68, 73–74
docosahexaenoic acid, 177
dust mites, 213–14
dyes, in skincare products, 102

E

Earth's Best, 186
Earth Science, 10
eczema, 103–8
Eczema Lotion, 106–7

eggplant, 32
electronic devices, 155–59, 161
endocrine disrupters, 6
Environmental Defense Fund, 34
environmentally-safe products, baby-safe products and, xviii–xx
Environmental Protection Agency, 7, 14, 19, 22, 23–24, 25, 30, 34
Equal artificial sweetener, 172
essential oils, 85
EWG, 30
exposure to toxins or poisons, 71, 76–77

F

fabric softeners, 86
fat-free foods, 170–71
first aid, 71
flame-retardant chemicals, 47–48, 150
flaxseed oil, 106
fleas, 215–16
flooring, 44–45
  cleaning products, 80–81, 89
floor polish, 67, 68
fluoride, 200–201
foaming and sudsy products, 111–14
food and diet
  allergies, 174–75
  avoiding infection from germs in, 38–40, 99
  baby food purees, 186–87
  baby-safe approach to, 163–64, 165, 176, 182–88, 202–3
  chemical additives, 170
  child's acceptance of, 194–96
  in day-care facilities, 99
  dining out, 197–200
  fat-free, 170–71
  fruits and vegetables, 30–33, 176–77
  gluten-free, 169
  homegrown vegetables, 242–44
  iPhone app for guidance on, 40
  locally-produced products, 166–67, 168
  multigrain products, 169
  during pregnancy, 29–41, 56–57
  probiotics in, 106
  raw foods diet, 168–69
  seafood, 33–36, 177, 178
  serving utensils and tableware, 190–92
  snacks and treats, 182–83, 185
  storing and reheating, 191–92
  teaching children about, 192–93
  terminology of food products, 164–74
Food and Drug Administration, 34, 173
Food and Water Watch, 26
formaldehyde, 8, 47, 51–52
fragrances and perfumes
  alcohol in, 68
  in disposable diapers, 121
  indoor air quality and, 19–22
  labeling, 7–8
  in laundry detergent, 85
  synthetic, 7–8, 12, 19
free-range animals, 172
Frontline, 215–16
furniture
  plastic, 131
  potential toxins in, 8, 51–52
  see also changing table; cribs and bassinets
Fuzbaby, 117

G
gardening, 242–44, 262
garlic oil, 249
gDiapers, 117
genetically modified organisms (GMOs), 173–74
glass cleaners, 65–66, 212
gluten-free foods, 169
GMOs. *see* genetically modified organisms
GoGo squeeZ, 186
GoodLight candles, 21
grapefruit, 32
grapes, 31
grass-fed animals, 171
Greenguard Certification Program, 51
Green Planet Paints, 42
Greenpoint Brands, 143
greens, 31
Green Sprouts, 191
Green Toys, 142
Guilt Trip, The, 114

H
haddock, 35
hair styling products, 7, 8, 13, 68
halibut, 35
hand washing
  basic baby-safe practices for, 97, 126–27
  by day-care staff, 98, 99
  importance of, 92, 95–96, 99
  outdoor play and, 238
  soaps and lotions, 7, 66, 68
  teaching children about, 93–94
  see also antibacterial and antimicrobial products
Happy Family Organic Superfoods, 186
Harmony Interior Acrylic Latex, 42
hazardous waste disposal, 70–72
heating system, air quality and, 17–18
HEPA air filters, 45
herbicides, 234
heterocyclic amines, 181, 182
high chairs, 131, 147–49
home maintenance
  for baby-safe environment, 54–55
  cleaning products, 60–72, 82–84, 88–90
  insect control in, 248–49
  see also bathroom, cleaning; indoor air quality; kitchen; nursery
hormone-free meats, 173
Hourglass cosmetics, 10
humidifiers, 105
hydrocortisone, 107–8
hydrogenated fats, 172
hydrogen peroxide, xix
hydroquinone, 8

I
IKEA, 51
Indestructibles, 143
indoor air quality, 14–21, 42–43, 45, 55–56, 80, 213–14
infections and communicable diseases
  hand washing to avoid, 79, 92, 95–96
  risk of, 96–97
  strategies for avoiding, 95–96, 97–101
  see also bacteria and germs
insect repellents. *see* pesticides and insecticides
insect stings and bites, 247–48
Integrated Pest Management, 249

International Fragrance Association, 20
itches and scratching, 106

J

Josie Maran Cosmetics, 10
Juice Beauty, 10
Juvenile Products Manufacturers Association, 50

K

kitchen
  baby-safe designs in, 193, 203
  cleaning for food prep, 187–89
  cleaning products, 72–74
  garbage, 248–49
  see also cooking
kiwi, 32
Korres, 10

L

labeling
  of art supplies, 135
  of fragrances and perfumes, 7–8
  of high chairs, 149
  of household cleaning products, 68–70
  iPhone app for evaluating, 69
  of organic products, 12, 165–67
  of personal care products, 113
  of strollers, 155
  terminology of foodstuffs, 168–74
  of toys and play gear, 130, 134–35, 160
latex, 121
laundry, 67, 85–87, 90, 104
lawn care, 232–38
lead contamination
  health threats from, 25–26, 133
  legal bans on, 132–33
  minimizing exposure to, 26
  in nursery, 43
  potential sources of, 25
  testing for, 43
  in toys, 132–33, 135
Lifefactory, 28
lip balm, 9, 256
lipstick, 7, 8, 9
listeria monocytogenes, 38, 39
litter box, 217
Little Partners Learning Tower, 192
locally-produced foods, 166–67, 168
Lullaby Paints, 42
lye, 66–67

M

mackerel, 35
magnets, 137
makeup, 11–14
mango butter, 110
mangoes, 32
mascara, 7
mattresses, 46–50
MEA, 112–13
meats, 39–40, 171–72, 173, 180–82
melanoma, 250
Melissa and Doug, 143
mercury, 34, 35–36, 37, 177
methylmercury. *see* mercury
microwave cooking, 191–92
milk, 39, 178–80
mineral oil, 102, 108–10, 250–51

Modern-Twist, 191
moisturizing agents, 105
monoethanolamine, 112–13
mosquitoes, 246–47
mouthwash, 68
multigrain foods, 169
mushrooms, 32
musical playthings, 138–39

N

nail care products, 7, 8, 13
National Institutes of Health, 69
National Research Council, 68
natural foods, 171
Natural Resources Defense Council, 27, 69
nectarines, 31
neem oil, 248–49
NeoNourish Complex, 107
noise exposure from toys, 138
nursery
  baby-safe approach to decorating, 41, 57
  bedding, 46–50
  changing table in, 50–52
  flooring and wall materials, 41–46
  windows, 51–52

O

oils, baby, 109–10
omega-3s, 34, 177, 178, 180, 207–8
100% Pure, 10
onions, 32
organic products
  bedding materials, 46, 48–49
  changing table materials, 51
  cosmetics, 12
  diapers, 116–17
  fresh produce, 30–33
  labeling of, 12, 165–67
  milk, 179
organophosphates, 233
outdoor space
  baby-safe approach to enjoying, 261–63
  decks and porches, 240–41
  furniture, 240
  lawns, 232–38
  play sets and structures, 240–42
  vegetable gardens, 242–44
oven cleaning products, 66–67
OXO Tot, 125
oxybenzone, 250, 252
oysters, 35

P

PABA, 252
pacifiers, 28
  cleaning, 72–74
paint
  nursery, 42–43
  recommended brands of, 42
  storing and disposing of, 71–72
pajamas, 47–48
papayas, 32
paper towels, 81
para-aminobenzoic acid, 252
parabens, 6
particle board, 8
pasteurized dairy products, 39
PBDEs, 47, 150

PCBs, 38
peaches, 31
peas, 32
peppers, 31
perfluorooctanoic acid, 189–90
perfumes. *see* fragrances and perfumes
personal care products
  labeling, 113
  potential toxins in, 6–9
  during pregnancy, caution in use of, 3–6
  shopping for and using, 9–14, 55
  see also cosmetics and skincare products
personal hygiene
  basic baby-safe practices for, 126–28
  bathing products, 111–14, 127
  outdoor play and, 238
  practices in day-care facilities, 98–100
  see also hand washing
pesticides and insecticides
  avoiding, 30–33
  for flea infestation, 216
  on grass, 232–38
  labeling, 173
  natural alternatives to, 244–47, 248–49, 262
  from neighboring properties, 236–37, 244
  organic food to avoid, 166
  potential health risks from, 30, 37, 232–34
  sources of, 37
  in sunscreen, 255
  use of, 249
petrochemicals, 9, 108–10
petroleum jelly, 108–9
pets
  allergic reactions to, 207
  babies and, 205–6
  baby-safe approach to living with, 228–29
  bathing, 207–10, 228
  brushing, 208
  controlling allergens of, 213–14
  fleas from, 215–16
  food, 226–27
  interactions with babies, 220–27
  shedding, 206–8, 210–11
  skin care for, 206–7
  sources of toxic exposure for, 210–12
  toys, 218–20
  wastes, 216–17
PFOA, 189–90
phthalates, 7, 12, 131–32
pineapples, 32
pistachios, 180
P'kolino, 144
PlanToys, 144
plants, indoor, 18
playgrounds, 241–42
Plum Organics, 186
pollack, 35
polyamine, 191
polybrominated diphenyl ethers, 47–48, 150
polychlorinated biphenyls, 38
polyethylene, 191
polypropylene, 191
polyurethane, 47
polyvinyl chloride, 131–32, 133, 134, 190–91
pool safety, 257–59
potatoes, 31
potty training, 116
powder, baby, 124–25

pregnancy
avoiding exposure to paints during, 42–43
avoiding food-borne bacteria in, 38–40
diet and nutrition during, 29–41, 56–57
indoor air quality and, 14, 16, 55–56
iPhone app for diet guidance during, 40
preparing pet for baby during, 220–21
sense of smell during, 19, 20
topical absorption of toxins during, 5
use of personal care products during, 3–14, 55
preservatives, 11, 170
Preserve Products, 191
probiotics, 106
PVC, 131–32

R

radon gas, 18
raw foods diet, 168–69
recycling code 7 materials, 28
Research Institute for Fragrance Materials, 20
restaurants, 197–200
Revolution pet medications, 215–16
Rogen, Seth, 114

S

saccharine, 172
Safe Drinking Water Act, 26
salmon, 35
sardines, 35
scallops, 35
screen time, 155–59, 161
seafood, 33–36, 39–40, 177, 178
Seafood Watch, 178
seed oils, 106–7
shampoos and conditioners
for babies, 111–13
for pets, 207–9
potential toxins in, 6, 7, 8, 67–68, 112–13
during pregnancy, 6, 7–8
shark, 35, 177
shaving gels, 6, 112–13
shea butter, 110
sheets and blankets, 48–49, 50
shower curtains, 131
shrimp, 35
sippy cups, 28
skin, baby's
addressing problems in, 103–8
basic baby-safe practices for, 127–28
diaper changes and care for, 125–26, 128
diaper rash on, 122–25
good products for care of, 102–3, 106–7, 110
potential toxins in products for, 102, 108–9
preventing itching, 106
protecting from sun exposure, 110–11, 249–57, 263
sensitivity of, 91–92, 101, 103
skin cancer risk, 249–50
smells, 19–22
of arts and crafts supplies, 135
of household cleaning products, 63–64
from pet waste, 217–18
smoke detectors, 18
soaps and cleansers
antimicrobial, 64–66, 68, 74–79, 100–101
baby-safe products and practices, 84–85, 88–90
baby's sensitivity to, 91–92
disposing of toxic products, 70–72

for floors, 80–81, 89
foaming and sudsy products for bathing, 111–14
household cleaning products to avoid, 60–70
kitchen, baby-safe products for, 72–74
labeling of, 68–70
laundry, 67, 85–86, 90, 104
mother's use of, during pregnancy, 6, 7
potential toxins in, 64–68
smell of, 63–64
see also personal hygiene
sodium hydroxide, 66–67
sodium hypochlorite. *see* bleach
sodium laureth sulfate, 67–68, 112
sodium lauryl sulfate, 67–68
solvents, 67
spinach, 31
Splenda, 172
spray tan solution, 6
squash, 31
steroid drugs, 107–8
stevia, 172
strawberries, 31
strollers, 131, 153–55
stuffed animals, 139, 214
sucralose, 172
sudden infant death syndrome, 50
Suki Skincare, 10
sulfates, 67–68
sunscreens and sunblocks, 110–11, 249–57, 263
superbugs, 66, 75
sushi, 39
swaddling, 50
Sweet'n Low, 172
sweet potatoes, 32
swimming pools, 257–59
swordfish, 35, 177

T

tap water, 23
TEA, 112–13
teaching children
computer electronics for, 156–57
food prep and cooking, 192–93
how to drink from a cup, 115
personal hygiene, 93–94
tilapia, 35
tile cleaning products, 66–67, 82
tilefish, 35
titanium dioxide, 250, 251
tofu, 180
toilet cleaners, 82
tomatoes, 31
toothpaste, 6, 66, 67–68, 200–201
topical absorption, 5
Toxic Substances Control Act, 61
toxoplasmosis, 216–17
toys and play gear
age-appropriate, 136
baby-safe choices for, 134–40, 160–61
battery-operated, 137–38
choking hazards, 136–37
cleaning, 142–46
musical, 138–39
noises from, 138
for pets, 218–20
plastic, 7, 28
potential toxins in, 130–34
recall notices, 145

toys and play gear (*continued*)
used, 141–42
warning labels on, 130
trans-fats, 172
triclorocarbon, 66
triclosan, 66, 75
triethanoamine, 112–13
Trifexis, 215–16
trout, 35
tub cleaners, 82–84
tuna, 35

U
ultraviolet light, 253
Under the Nile, 117, 144
used goods
car seats, 152–53
toys, 141–42
UVA/UVB, 253

V
vacuuming, 45, 213–14
Vectra, 215–16
vegan diet, 168
vegetable oils, 110
vinegar, 84–85
vision, child's, 158–59
vitamin D, 178
volatile organic compounds, 14
in flooring materials, 44
health risks of, 47
in paints, 42–43
sources of, 46
Vulli, 144

W
walls, nursery, 42–43
water
bathwater, 114–15
bottled, 26–28
child's intake of, 22
good practices for ensuring safety of, 22–25, 56
potential toxins in, 25–26
from refrigerator, 24–25
testing, 23–24
weed killing chemicals, 234
whitefish, 35
Whole Foods, 68
windows, 51–52
wipes, baby, 125–26, 128
wood
cutting boards, 188–89
outdoor structures and furniture, 240–41
pressure-treated, 240, 244
toys, 136

Y
YOLO Colorhouse, 42

Z
zinc dioxide, 250, 251

About the Authors

Kevin Schwartz, babyganics CEO (Tyler & Ryan's dad)

It was in the early 2000s that I got really serious about creating a baby-focused consumer products company and the babyganics brand. Starting a business is tough, for sure, but it's a lot easier with a guiding mission. Mine was to develop the kind of household and personal care products that would help other parents create a baby-safe environment so that their babies would be free to explore and develop their minds and bodies. Babyganics was born out of the instinct we have as parents to give our babies the absolute best chance to become amazing at every age.

I'm a Long Islander, born and raised, and have been able to establish the company close to home where I have a huge crew of family and lifelong friends. When I'm not in the office, I'm either helping Tyler perfect his football tackle, making music with Ryan, or taking a long run with my wife (and the jogging strollers!).

Keith Garber, babyganics President (Zach, Skylar & Ashton's dad)

I joined Kevin at babyganics because we share a very similar vision of a baby-safe world and the kind of products that can help parents create it. My goal is to help make sure that all the great products we develop are available in as many places that parents shop as possible. That's why I find myself on the road all over the country. But my favorite place to travel to is home, to be with my family.

I also live on Long Island, not too far from Kevin. When I'm not on the sidelines coaching Zach's soccer team, I might be helping teach Ashton to crawl, or having a tea party with Skylar and my wife!

Kevin and Keith often speak on topics related to safety and sustainability. Everywhere they go, they find parents who are hungry for information about the dangers of potentially harmful chemicals and toxins, and are looking for smart and effective solutions. Kevin and Keith are both thrilled and rewarded to be able to offer their help and expertise.